Smell and Taste Complaints

THE MOST COMMON COMPLAINTS SERIES

Headache
Egilius L. H. Spierings

Confusion
Karl E. Misulis and Terri Edwards-Lee

Neck Complaints
Michael Ronthal

Chest Pain
Richard C. Becker

Gait Disorders
Michael Ronthal

Smell and Taste Complaints

**Christopher H. Hawkes, B.Sc., M.D.,
F.C.R.P.(Ed.), F.R.C.P.(Lond.)**

*Consultant Neurologist, Essex Neuroscience Centre,
Oldchurch Hospital, Romford, Essex, England;
Honorary Consultant and Lecturer in Clinical Neurology,
The National Hospital for Neurology and Neurosurgery
and Institute of Neurology, Queen Square, London*

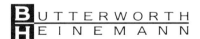

An imprint of Elsevier Science

Amsterdam   Boston   London   New York   Oxford   Paris
San Diego   San Francisco   Singapore   Sydney   Tokyo

Butterworth–Heinemann is an imprint of Elsevier Science.

Every effort has been made to ensure that the drug dosage schedules within this text are accurate and conform to standards accepted at time of publication. However, as treatment recommendations vary in the light of continuing research and clinical experience, the reader is advised to verify drug dosage schedules herein with information found on product information sheets. This is especially true in cases of new or infrequently used drugs.

Recognizing the importance of preserving what has been written, Elsevier Science prints its books on acid-free paper whenever possible.

Library of Congress Cataloging-in-Publication Data

Hawkes, Christopher H.
    Smell and taste complaints / Christopher H. Hawkes.
      p. ; cm. — (The most common complaints series)
    Includes bibliographical references and index.
    ISBN 0-7506-7287-0) (pbk. : alk. paper)
    1. Smell disorders. 2. Taste disorders. I. Title. II. Series.
    [DNLM: 1. Olfaction Disorders. 2. Taste Disorders. WV 301 H392d 2002]
    RF341 .H39 2002
    616.8'7—dc21

                                          2001058613

British Library Cataloguing-in-Publication Data
A catalogue record for this book is available from the British Library.

The publisher offers special discounts on bulk orders of this book.
For information, please contact:

    Manager of Special Sales
    Elsevier Science
    225 Wildwood Avenue
    Woburn, MA 01801-2041
    Tel: 781-904-2500
    Fax: 781-904-2620

For information on all Butterworth–Heinemann publications available, contact our World Wide Web home page at: http://www.bh.com

10 9 8 7 6 5 4 3 2 1

Printed in the United States of America

Contents

Preface

It is common practice to lump smell and taste sensations together. This is an anachronism as the two modalities develop individually from an embryological standpoint and are almost completely separate in the brain at the subcortical level. Phylogenetically olfaction developed first; taste is a relatively new thalamic-dependent feature. The fact that so many patients confuse smell and taste should not permit their assimilation by clinicians.

According to Hoffman and coworkers, there are at least 2.7 million (1.4%) Americans with some form of chronic olfactory dysfunction. Most clinicians rarely bother to ask about or test patients for smell disorders, an approach that reflects partly in the relative lack of importance attached by many patients to olfaction, and partly in the lack of diagnostically useful clinical information obtained. All this, coupled with inappropriate, often encrusted, smell test kits, has ensured that the smell sense is often ignored. Such an approach is wrong; for example, anosmia has always been of considerable medicolegal importance, commanding major awards in head-injured patients particularly if their profession depends on a good sense of smell. Furthermore, defective smell sense has been recently identified as an early phenomenon in Parkinson's and Alzheimer's diseases so that in scientific circles, at least, olfaction is now back on the map.

The situation with taste is even more fraught. In the Hoffman survey an estimated 1.1 million (0.6%) suffered some form of taste disturbance. Clinicians might occasionally ask about taste loss in someone with a facial palsy but that is where taste examination ends. Formal taste testing is studiously ignored in the clinical setting, as there are few diseases where their diagnosis may be advanced. I suspect this is an attitude borne out of our current ignorance and there is a vast amount of scientific information awaiting discovery that might provide important clues in unraveling diseases.

C.H.H.

Hoffman HJ, Ishii EK, MacTurk RH. Age-related changes in the prevalence of smell/taste problems among the United States adult population. Results of the 1994 disability supplement to the National Health Interview Survey (NHIS). Ann N Y Acad Sci. 1998; 855:716–722.

Acknowledgments

I would like to express my deep indebtedness for the help and support I have received on numerous occasions from Professor Gerd Kobal, University of Erlangen, Germany, who first stimulated my interest in chemosensory function.

I am also indebted to the following individuals for advice and guidance in preparation of this work: Dr. Thomas Hummel, University of Dresden, Germany; Dr. Glenis Scadding, Royal National TNE Hospital, London; and Mr. Hashem Kaddour, Harold Wood Hospital, Essex.

I am most grateful for the Medical Photography Unit at Oldchurch Hospital for their painstaking work.

Finally, I wish to thank my wife, Mahboub, and children, Elizabeth and Catherine, for their tolerance while I wrote this book.

Smell and Taste Complaints

Olfaction

Anatomy and Physiology of Smell Sense

ANATOMY

It must first be emphasized that there are two noses (right and left) and each has a triple innervation—the trigeminal sensory nerves, the olfactory nerves, and the autonomic supply. The trigeminal component supplies the vast majority of the inner mucosal lining of the nose with perception of touch, temperature, pain, tickle, and itching. Most odorous compounds stimulate all three nerves in varying proportions. Vanillin, for example, is one of few specific olfactory stimulants whereas ammonia has powerful trigeminal and olfactory components. It has been suggested that the trigeminal nerve contributes partially to smell appreciation but the issue has never been fully resolved. Certainly anosmics can detect "impure" smells, that is, those with a trigeminal component such as menthol or camphor.

The olfactory receptor area is small and located high in the nasal cavity in the upper septal zone, cribriform plate, medial wall of the superior, and to a lesser extent middle turbinate (Figure 1-1). The radiological anatomy is shown in Figure 1-2. Histologically the olfactory epithelium consists of a sheet of supporting cells with interspersed olfactory neurons that form knob-like protrusions above the level of the supporting cells (Figure 1-3). The olfactory knobs have 3–50 ciliary processes that contain receptor cells. They form tight junctions with adjacent supporting cells and openings of Bowman's glands. Bowman's glands secrete mucus essential for olfactory analysis. It contains a protein called olfactory binding protein that binds to odorant molecules and assists in transmitting the odorant to membrane proteins within the cell membrane of the olfactory dendrite and supporting cells.

Olfactory analysis has to take place in a fluid environment. There are an estimated 12 million olfactory receptor cells in the human but this number is dwarfed by approximately 4 billion (10^9) in the equivalent canine area. The axons of the bipolar olfactory cells are incredibly small at 0.2μ diameter making them among the thinnest in the nervous

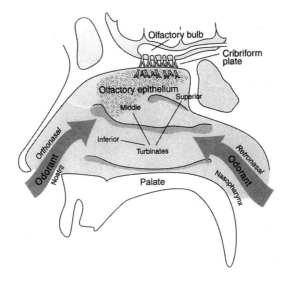

Figure 1-1. Anatomy of olfactory area and connections. Note that the olfactory epithelium extends over the middle turbinate. Volatile chemicals can reach the sensory epithelium via the nares or via the pharynx during chewing or swallowing, for example. (Reprinted with permission from Rawson N. The neurobiology of taste and smell. In TE Finger, WL Silver, D Restrepo (eds), Human Olfaction. New York: Wiley-Liss, 2000; Chapter 11.)

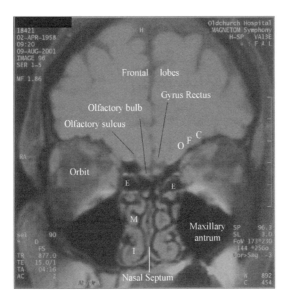

Figure 1-2. MRI scan (coronal T1 weighted) in healthy 45-year-old woman showing frontal lobes, orbits, olfactory bulbs, olfactory sulcus, and gyrus rectus. OFC is the orbitofrontal cortex. Letter "E" indicates part of the ethmoid sinuses that are frequently honeycomb structures. Letter "I" is the right inferior turbinate; "M" is the right middle turbinate. The superior turbinate and infundibulum are not clearly shown due to the posterior coronal section.

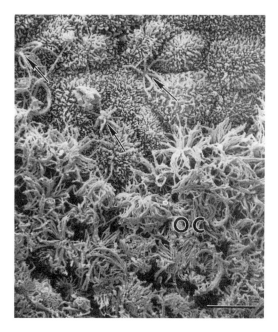

Figure 1-3. Scanning electron micrograph of olfactory mucosal surface. Olfactory region lacks the dense cilia covering, and dendritic knobs (arrows) can be seen between microvilli-covered supporting cells. The adjacent area has a dense covering of sensory olfactory cilia (OC). Bar = 5μ. (Reprinted with permission from Morrison EE, Moran DT. Anatomy and ultrastructure of the human olfactory neuroepithelium. In RL Doty (ed), Handbook of Olfaction and Gustation. New York: Marcel Dekker Inc., 1995; Figure 3-10.)

system and consequently they conduct slowly at about 1 meter/second. Groups of these non-myelinated axons are enclosed in one sleeve of a neurolemmal cell; hence axons are virtually in direct contact with each other (a gap of only 100 Å) and cross talk between these axons is possible.

Apart from cochlear neurons, the olfactory neurons are the only ones in the central nervous system that are capable of regeneration and they are continually turning over. There are no data for humans but it is estimated from animal work that they live for about 35 days. This point probably reflects their ancient origins, but on a more practical level explains why a few people with, for example, post-traumatic anosmia may eventually recover.

The general somatic nerve supply to the nose derives from branches of the trigeminal nerve. The anterior and posterior ethmoid nerves, which are branches of the nasociliary nerve (ophthalmic division of V), supply the upper part of the nasal cavity (Figures 1-4 and 1-5). The posterior part of the nasal cavity is fed by the nasopalatine nerve, which is a branch of the maxillary nerve. Autonomic supply to the nose comes from the sphenopalatine ganglion. Vascular disturbance in this ganglion is said to cause a form of facial pain associated with nasal congestion known as sphenopalatine neuralgia. It

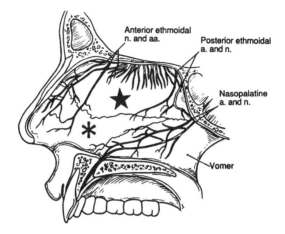

Figure 1-4. Sagittal view of nasal septum showing arteries and nerve supply. The black star represents the perpendicular plate of the ethmoid. The asterisk indicates the quadrangular cartilage and approximate position of the vomeronasal organ. (Reprinted with permission from Lanza DC, Kennedy DW, Koltai PJ. Applied nasal anatomy and embryology. ENT Journal 1991;70;416–422.)

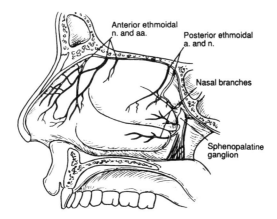

Figure 1-5. Sagittal view of lateral nasal wall showing arteries and nerve supply. (Reprinted with permission from Lanza DC, Kennedy DW, Koltai PJ. Applied nasal anatomy and embryology. Ear Nose and Throat Journal 1991;70;416–422.)

can be abolished sometimes by applying cocaine to the ganglion.

The nasal cavity is supplied with blood by tributaries of the external and internal carotid arteries. The ophthalmic branch of the internal carotid artery gives rise to the anterior and posterior ethmoidal arteries which supply the upper part of the nasal cavity (see Figures 1-4 and 1-5). The sphenopalatine artery, also derived from the internal carotid, feeds the posterior nasal cavity. The anterior nose is fed by branches of the facial and internal maxillary arteries that derive from the external carotid artery. Theoretically, impaired blood supply in the ethmoidal arteries could interfere with olfaction but this has not been described in practice, probably because of good collateral supply. Laser-Doppler flowmeter measurement in the human nasal respiratory epithelium yields a high rate at about 42ml/100g/minute. This is probably required to allow toxins in the bloodstream to come in contact with xenobiotic metabolizing enzymes. There are no data on human olfactory epithelial blood flow but this is likely to be high as it is in animals.

The anatomy of the bulb is complex and is shown diagrammatically in Figures 1-6 and 1-7 and Color Plate 1, along with some of its 20 or more known neurotransmitters. It should be noted that axons of the olfactory cells make contact with the dendrites of mitral and tufted cells (i.e., axo-dendritic synapses) and in so doing form curious looking clumps called glomeruli. There are only 12,000 glomeruli available to handle messages from 12 million olfactory axons (i.e., 1000:1 convergence ratio). Impulses next pass along the olfactory tracts that lie on the undersurface of the frontal lobes. Some fibers project back to the contralateral olfactory bulb (Figure 1-6A).

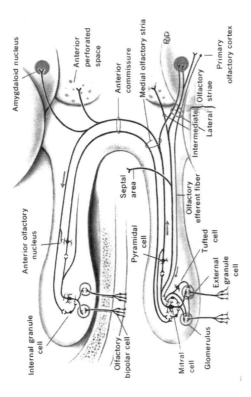

Figure 1-6. A. Anatomy of the olfactory bulbs and the 3 major divisions connecting to the brain.

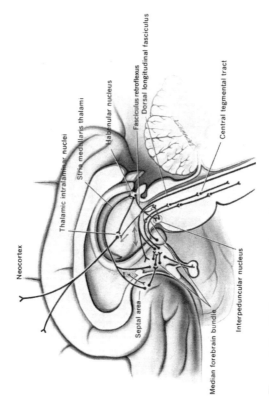

Figure 1-6. B, Some connections of the limbic system and septal area.

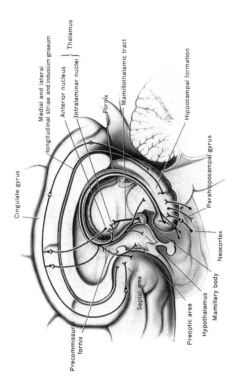

Figure 1-6. **C,** The "Papez circuit": hippocampus via fornix to mamillary body; via mamillothalamic tract to anterior nuclear group of thalamus; via cingulate gyrus to hippocampus.

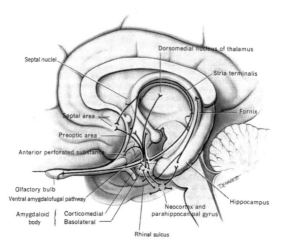

Figure 1-6. **D**, Connections of the limbic system and amygdaloid body. (Reprinted with permission from Noback CR, Demarest RJ. The Human Nervous System (3rd ed). Boston: McGraw-Hill, 1981; Chapter 15.)

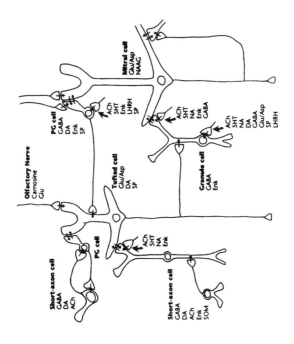

Figure 1-7. Anatomy of the bulb and some of its neurotransmitters. ACh, acetylcholine; DA, dopamine; DLH, DL-homocysteate; Enk, Met-enkephalin; GABA, gamma-aminobutyric acid; Glu/Asp, glutamate or aspartate; 5HT, 5-hydroxytryptamine; LHRH, luteinizing-hormone-releasing hormone; NA, noradrenaline; NAAG, *N*-acetyl-aspartyl-glutamate; SOM, somatostatin; SP, substance P; PG cell, periglomerular cell. Small arrows show direction of synaptic transmission; solid arrows indicate centrifugal inputs to the olfactory bulb. (Reprinted with permission from Kratskin IL. Functional anatomy, central connections and neurochemistry of the mammalian olfactory bulb. In RL Doty (ed), Handbook of Olfaction and Gustation. New York: Marcel Dekker Inc., 1995; Figure 4-6.)

The central connections are complex, but basically split in three directions:

1. *Septal area* and from there via the stria medullaris to the habenular nucleus, thalamic intralaminar nuclei, and interpeduncular nucleus (Figure 1-6B). Another branch from the septal area connects via the cingulate gyrus to the hippocampal formation that is part of the limbic system (Figure 1-6C).
2. *Amygdaloid nucleus* (Figure 1-6D). Connections from here go to and from the neocortex and parahippocampal gyrus; dorsomedial nucleus of thalamus; preoptic and septal areas.
3. *Primary olfactory cortex* that is medially situated within the temporal lobe and consists of
    a. The prepyriform cortex, an area adjacent to the lateral olfactory stria (see Figure 1-6A) and the rostral part of the uncus.
    b. Limen insulae and uncus, sometimes called the intermediate pyriform cortex. The limen insulae is a tongue of cortex just medial to the anterior perforated substance (see Figure 1-6A) and the uncus is a hook-like structure when viewed from below, situated deeply and medially within the temporal lobe, continuous laterally with the amygdaloid body. There are important connec-

tions from the primary olfactory cortex to the orbitofrontal cortex (see Figure 1-2), which is probably an association area concerned with smell identification and discrimination (qv). Cortical areas that are directly concerned with smell appreciation when stimulated consist only of the prepyriform and intermediate pyriform cortex.

What is unusual is the fact that most impulses reach the cerebral cortex without first relaying through the thalamus unlike all other sensory modalities including taste. This fact emphasizes the primitive origins of the rhinencephalon that evolved long before other sensory paths that all relay in the thalamus. Some have suggested that the olfactory bulb is in fact the equivalent of the thalamus but it seems likely that olfactory signals do reach the thalamus (mediodorsal nucleus) where they interact with trigeminal afferents.

VOMERONASAL ORGAN (JACOBSON'S ORGAN) AND NERVUS INTERMEDIUS

Although the existence of the vomeronasal organ (VNO) in animals is undisputed, there is doubt regarding the human counterpart. In the developing human fetus there appears to be a VNO that stains for luteinizing hormone releasing hormone (LHRH), but its connections with the olfactory bulb disappear or become displaced and hard to locate at about 19 weeks of age. In adults a VNO exists bilaterally on the anterior third of the nasal septum and opens through a pit about 1–2 cm back from the posterior margin of the nostril (see Figure 1.4). Some claim the VNO is present in all healthy humans, others say what is observed is just a vestige. Structurally the cells of VNO are similar to olfactory epithelial cells and immune stains show reaction to neuron-specific enolase and a protein gene product (PGP-9.5), which typifies neurons and neuroendocrine cells. However, they do not react to olfactory marker protein like all olfactory neurons.

It is suggested that the VNO is a receptor for pheromones such as androstenone that control sexual behavior. It is also held that pheromones cause menstrual synchrony, improved mood, and relaxation, all of which act possibly through the VNO. Application of steroids to this region has been claimed to produce changes in mood, autonomic function, and hormone levels but the results are disputed. A receptor potential can be elicited from the VNO and shown to be more responsive to pheromones than the nearby olfactory epithelium. A neural connection to the brain (vomeronasal nerve; Figure 1-8) is observed up to the 8th month

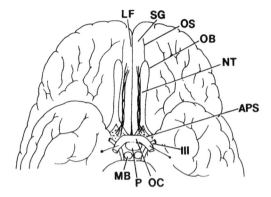

Figure 1-8. Outline of the ventral surface of the human frontal and temporal lobes to show the position of the intracranial portion of the nervus intermedius. FP = longitudinal fissure; SG = straight gyrus; OS = olfactory sulcus; OB = olfactory bulb; NT = nervus terminalis; APS = anterior perforated substance; III = oculomotor nerve; OC = optic chiasm; P = pituitary gland; MB = mamillary body. (Reprinted with permission from Schwanzel-Fukuda M, Pfaff DW. Structure and function of the nervus terminalis. In RL Doty (ed), Handbook of Olfaction and Gustation. New York: Marcel Dekker Inc., 1995; Figure 38-2.)

of human fetal life but it has not yet been demonstrated in adults. Another nerve seen easily in animals, probably separate from the vomeronasal nerve, and claimed to exist in adult humans is the nervus terminalis or "zeroeth" cranial nerve. It also arises from the VNO but projects directly to the septal and preoptic areas of the brain (see Figure 1-8). This is a unique property in that it enters the brain without relaying in either the thalamus or olfactory bulb. This could provide a route for toxic substances to enter the brain unimpeded. Unlike the olfactory nerve, the nervus terminalis has LHRH activity and is a structure separate from the vomeronasal nerve. Its function awaits clarification but it is doubtless concerned with chemoreception.

In summary, odors make contact with the olfactory area located high in the nasal cavity. The estimated 12 million human receptor cells converge upon much fewer cells in the olfactory bulb. From here the major connections spread out in three directions—to the septal area, amygdaloid nucleus, and primary olfactory cortex and from the latter to the orbitofrontal cortex. Subsequent connections involve the hypothalamus, thalamus, hippocampus, and basal ganglia. In principle, the olfactory pathways may thereafter connect to any region in the nervous system; hence a noxious substance (virus, chemical) may go virtually wherever it wants.

PHYSIOLOGY

During normal inspiration 5–10% of the air reaches the olfactory receptors but the act of sniffing redirects 20% of the air (approximately 250 ml) from its usual mainly horizontal path, upwards to the olfactory cleft. The frequency with which animals and humans sniff would suggest that this maneuver enhances odor analysis and detection, although experimentally this has been hard to prove. An important function of the nose is to warm and humidify incoming air because this facilitates olfaction. The nose filters potentially harmful particles, but even more significant and not widely appreciated is the amazing ability of the nasal mucosa to detoxify incoming chemicals—a function surpassed only by the liver. The nasal mucosa possesses a considerable amount of cytochrome P-450-dependent mono-oxygenase activity that allows them to detoxify a variety of drugs and harmful xenobiotics.

Surprisingly, only one nostril is ever fully patent at a time in 80% of healthy people, and this will vary throughout the day—the "nasal cycle." The precise reason for this apparent economy is not well understood but it has to be taken into account when testing smell sense unilaterally.

The human nose, contrary to popular belief, can detect certain chemicals at extremely low concentration. For example methoxy-isobutylpyrazine (musty) may be detected in a concentration of 0.0002 parts per billion (ppb,v/v) and those not congenitally anosmic to it may detect androstenone (urinous) at a concentration of 0.2 ppb.

It is estimated that there are about 1000 human olfactory receptor genes but most, around 70%, are pseudogenes (i.e., they have no function). This contrasts with the rodent with only 5% pseudogenes and confirms that olfaction has become less important in the course of primate evolution. The human olfactory receptor gene family is distributed over several chromosomes. Zozulya and colleagues identified 347 putative functional receptor genes widely dispersed on all but 6 chromosomes, with the majority (155) on chromosome 11 and most of the others on chromosomes 1, 9, and 6.

Binding of an odor takes place on the ciliary process of the olfactory cell (Figure 1-9). This triggers a G-protein (GTP-binding regulatory protein) mediated increase in second messenger (cyclic adenosine monophosphate [cAMP]) derived from adenosine triphosphate (ATP). Cyclic AMP and probably other second messengers such as inositol triphosphate (IP3) activate ion channels to control the flow of sodium and calcium across the ciliary membrane. This amplifying cascade then probably causes opening of calcium-activated chloride channels and generation of an action potential. This potential can be recorded from the surface of the olfactory epithelium and is of remarkably slow duration—100–200 milliseconds or more.

CODING OF OLFACTORY INFORMATION

According to the stereochemical theory proposed by Amoore, smell differentiation relates to variation in molecular shape of the odor in question, which "locks" onto and activates specific receptor sites on olfactory neurons. Unfortunately this does not predict how all chemicals smell: some structurally different chemicals smell the same but others that are just stereoisomers smell quite different (Figure 1-10). There is good evidence of specific pheromone receptors located in the antennae of insects (e.g., the silk moth) where receptors for sex pheromones are highly tuned to particular isomers of the active compounds. These cells coexist with broadly tuned receptors. In the human olfactory epithelium, receptor cells sensitive to a particular odor respond to stimuli by variation of discharge frequency rate according to odor concentration. However, it appears that all receptor cells respond in varying degree to the majority of odorants irrespective of their physicochemical properties. It is

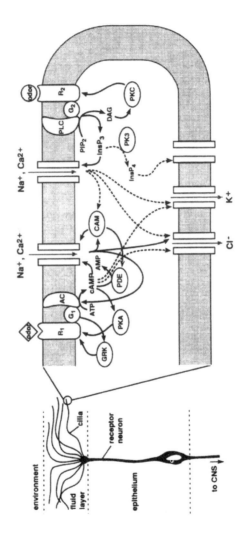

26

Figure 1-9. Pathways implicated in olfactory transduction. On the left is depicted the best understood pathway that involves a receptor protein (R_1), a GTP-binding protein (G_1), an adenylyl cyclase (AC) that produces adenosine cyclic monophosphate (cAMP), and a cation channel that is gated directly by cAMP. On the right is shown the inositol triphosphate pathway ($InsP_3$ or IP_3) for which the evidence in humans is less secure. The primary transduction pathways can target secondary ion channels of which the best known is a calcium-activated chloride channel— see lower part of drawing. Solid lines represent the better established pathways. Dashed lines are proposed pathways. PLC = a phospholipase C; DAG = diacylglycerol; G_2 = GTP-binding protein; GRK = G-protein coupled receptor kinase; PDE = phosphodiesterase; PKA & PKC = phosphokinases A and C; CAM = calcium calmodulin; $InsP_4$ = inositol tetrakisphosphate. (Reprinted with permission from Tache BW, Restrepo D. The neurobiology of taste and smell. In TE Finger, WL Silver, D Restrepo (eds), Olfactory Transduction. New York: Wiley-Liss, 2000; Chapter 7.)

27

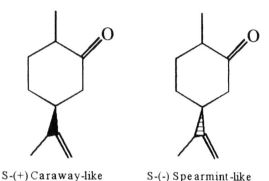

S-(+) Caraway-like   S-(-) Spearmint-like

Figure 1-10. Stereoisomers that have completely different smells.

surmised that receptor cells have varying sensitivities and that a "population" pattern is generated from many cells with similar sensitivity. Neurons that are activated by an individual smell or class of smells have not yet been found in humans.

A slightly different and speculative approach is taken by Freeman, who suggests that perception of odors depends on the simultaneous cooperative activity of millions of neurons spread throughout wide areas of the cortex. He proposes that every neuron in the olfactory bulb participates in generating each olfactory perception. The information is said to be carried by 40 Hz electrical rhythms called gamma waves. Information is thought to be transmitted not by waveform but by the amplitude pattern across the entire olfactory cortex. This pattern of gamma wave activity is generated by a unique nerve cell assembly that functions according to the principles of mathematical chaos.

It will be recalled that there are 12 million olfactory neurons in the human nose but only 12,000 glomeruli. Such 1000:1 convergence probably amplifies the signal but at the same time there is bound to be some distortion or loss of information; furthermore each glomerulus is in contact with the dendrites of many mitral and tufted cells (i.e., divergence of signal; see Color Plate 1). The latter cells are involved in complex reverberating circuits that allow positive and negative feedback. For example, mitral cells can modulate their own output by stimulating the granule cells that are inhibitory to them or by stimulating the excitatory inputs within the external plexiform layer. It is thought that reciprocal inhibition between neighboring mitral or tufted cells causes sharpened contrast between adjacent channels, similar to that known to occur in visual and common sensory pathways.

Experiments in the rat by Pinching and Døving suggest that there is a topographic arrangement in the bulb according to odor class. In the olfactory cortex there are small areas that receive input from large areas of the bulb; conversely large areas of olfactory cortex receive signals from small areas of the bulb.

It should be clear by now that the process of signal transmission to the brain is poorly understood, highly complex, and capable of considerable distortion en route. One is reminded of the early debates regarding receptor specificity for common sensation. Some considered spatial frequency analysis to be a sufficient means of encoding the signal but others claimed there were specific receptors. The situation only became fully resolved when electron microscope studies clearly showed specific receptors were present. Hence tuned olfactory receptors probably do exist in humans as in insects—it is a matter of finding them.

A transient decrease or loss of smell perception will occur for varying periods following odor exposure due to receptor "fatigue." For example, continuous inhalation of lemon or orange vapors can result in complete loss of smell sense for up to 11 minutes in healthy people. Although fatigue depends primarily on the duration and concentration of odor, certain compounds are more conducive to fatigue than others (e.g., vanillin that is notorious in this respect).

Unlike the eye and ear, the ability to localize and lateralize olfactory signals is poorly developed.

Unless the head can be moved it appears to be impossible to perceive the position of an odor. If the signal is introduced directly into the nostril, it may be lateralized only if the odor has some coexisting trigeminal component (e.g., menthol). Kobal and colleagues clearly showed that a specific olfactory stimulant such as vanillin could not be lateralized.

There are interesting differences in transmission of odors according to their hedonic properties. For example, it has been shown that responses to unpleasant odors such as menthol, acetaldehyde, and hydrogen sulphide elicit a cerebral evoked response of shorter latency and smaller amplitude upon stimulating the left nostril compared with the right nostril. Stimulation with the more pleasant vanillin or phenyl-ethyl-alcohol (rose-like) evokes potentials of shorter latency and smaller amplitude when the right nostril is activated compared to the left. Others report that pleasant emotions are mainly represented in the left cerebral hemisphere and unpleasant on the right side. Because the major cortical projection from one nostril is unilateral it may be argued that the higher amplitude later response on the left is the one for hedonic analysis. This would appear logical in that it allows more pleasant odors to be savored and examined at leisure. The unpleasant odors project more rapidly to the left side also, but the right/left latency differences are small, suggesting that bilateral cerebral activation is occurring—a useful way of activating a defensive motor response perhaps.

Lesions of the amygdalo-hypothalamic pathways impair odor and taste aversions, odor preference learning, and odor-mediated aspects of reproduction, suggesting a major role in feeding and neuroendocrine function at least for animals.

There is clinical evidence that medial bilateral temporal lobe lesions interfere with smell sense but only the ability to identify or discriminate smells correctly is lost and not odor detection. Removal of either temporal lobe results in significant reduction of olfactory discrimination ipsilateral to the side of nasal stimulation. Impairment is also seen ipsilaterally with removal of either frontal lobe, but if the right frontal lobe is removed (including the orbitofrontal cortex), discriminatory loss affects both nostrils. These ablation-type experiments have now been confirmed elegantly by functional brain mapping (see Color Plate 2). Hence the right orbitofrontal cortex that receives signals from both temporal lobes appears to be dominant for higher olfactory analysis.

Specific Anosmia

Some people are born unable to smell anything (congenital anosmia) while others cannot detect certain odors but their smell sense is otherwise normal.

This is termed specific anosmia or smell blindness and is analogous to color blindness. There are over 76 types of specific anosmias but the commoner ones are listed in Table 1-1 and their molecular structure in Figure 1-11. It can be seen that according to this survey almost half the healthy population are unable to detect androstenone. This compound has a sweaty or urinous odor and is suspected to have aphrodisiac properties in animals and humans. Interestingly, people who are initially anosmic to androsterone can improve their perception after training. Because of the frequency of smell

Table 1-1. Compounds associated with specific anosmia

Compound	Odor Quality	Percent Anosmic
Androstenone	Sweaty/urinous	47
Isobutyraldehyde	Malty	36
Cineole	Camphorous	33
Pyrroline	Spermous	12
Pentadecalactone	Musky	12
Carvone	Minty	8
Trimethylamine	Fishy	6
Isovaleric acid	Sweaty	3

Adapted from Wysocki CJ, Beauchamp GK. Individual differences in human olfaction. In CJ Wysocki, MR Kare (eds), Chemical Senses, Volume 3. Genetics of Perception and Communication. New York: Marcel Dekker Inc., 1991;353–373.

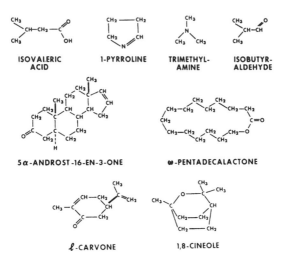

Figure 1-11. Structural formulae of the 8 proposed primary odors. (Reprinted with permission from Amoore JE, Steinle S. A graphic history of specific anosmia. In CJ Wysocki, MR Kare (eds), Chemical Senses, Volume 3. Genetics of Perception and Communication. New York: Marcel Dekker Inc., 1991; Figure 23-8.)

blindness it is probable that very few of us have a perfect sense of smell and that we all perceive a complex multicomponent aroma such as coffee or perfume in slightly different fashion. Smell blindness is probably inherited but the genetic mechanism for most compounds is poorly understood. Exalotide is a musky odor that cannot be detected by 12% of otherwise healthy people. The inability to detect this is thought to be inherited as an autosomal recessive trait but the genetics for androstenone are more complex and possibly X-linked.

Blind Smell

Sobel and colleagues coined this term, which has to be carefully distinguished from "smell blindness." Basically it implies detection of an odor by the brain in the absence of conscious perception. To demonstrate this, functional magnetic resonance imaging (fMRI) was used to localize brain activation induced by high and low concentrations of oestratetraenyl acetate. This is a putative human pheromone with a "chemical-like" odor. Although subjects reported verbally that they were unable to detect either concentration, their forced choice guess was better than chance for the higher concentration and both concentrations produced significant brain activation on fMRI, mainly in the right orbitofrontal cortex. In other words these subjects were able to detect odor at a subconscious level, without being fully aware that they could do so. These observations complement earlier work on "blind sight" where a subject correctly localizes objects although they cannot be seen consciously.

In summary, the initial act of sniffing directs odor molecules to the olfactory area where they become bound to the olfactory cilia. Complex reactions within the cilia result in signal amplification and generation of the action potential. Coding of olfactory information may depend on molecular shape or variation in discharge frequency in the olfactory nerve but the final signal in the temporal lobe is likely to be considerably modified. Further alterations in signal detection relate to receptor fatigue. Unlike the eye and ear, specific olfactory signals cannot be lateralized by healthy subjects unless there is a trigeminal component. There appear to be inter-hemispheric differences in processing according to the hedonic properties of odors, with pleasant aromas analyzed on the left, unpleasant on the right. The temporal lobes and particularly the right orbitofrontal cortex are involved in identifying and describing odors. Finally, many people are born with specific anosmia particularly to androstenone, isobutyraldehyde, and cineole and therefore will be exposed to a different olfactory environment than others.

INFLUENCES ON OLFACTION

Age, Gender, and Smoking

The effect of aging on olfactory ability in all aspects after the sixth decade is well documented. Aging influences odor perception at a later time in females and elderly women score higher on UPSIT (University of Pennsylvania Smell Identification Test) than men of the same age. Women are found to outperform men on most psychophysical tests but the effects are not marked. Tobacco smoking has less effect and relates to the quantity smoked. A very heavy smoker may have an UPSIT-40 score up to 4 points lower than a nonsmoker but cessation from smoking causes a gradual improvement of smell function.

Odor Memory and Analysis

Arousal is probably required for an odor to be remembered. Unless a situation involves deliberate smell analysis (such as wine or perfume sampling) exposure to odors is usually passive, but there is evidence that sleeping newborn babies (and adults) may respond to odors apparently without waking up. Several types of odor memories have been described, including long and short term, that are comparable to short- and long-term verbal memory. Short-term (working) memory for smell is the continual process of environmental monitoring for changes in background odor quality. It is probably a variant of short-term recall as any change in background odor can be perceived only with respect to smell signals recalled before the change took place.

Enhancement of olfactory memory by training is an undisputed faculty. Furthermore, training can alter smell sensitivity. Wysocki and colleagues showed that repeated exposure to androstenone over a period of 6 weeks caused substantial improvement of threshold in 10 of a group of 20 people initially unable to detect its odor. It is estimated that the average human can identify 2,000–4,000 different odors but with practice the skilled perfumer may increase this repertoire to 10,000. Such skill is not achieved without considerable training. There is, in fact, a grave deficiency of suitable descriptive language for the untrained person, many of whom find it difficult to attach words to smell. It is speculated that this may relate to relatively poor connections between the language centers of the brain (located in the precentral gyrus of the frontal lobe and superior temporal gyri) and olfactory areas.

There have been two recent attempts to overcome the problem of categorization: odor profiling and multidimensional scaling. Odor profiling attempts to characterize aromas by profiles of their individual qualities. A panel of experienced and specifically trained individuals learn a large number of reference standards and by consensus decide on appropriate descriptive terms. Average magnitude estimates are derived for various qualities such as intensity, pleasantness, unpleasantness, and familiarity.

Clearly such an approach is subjective and dependent on semantic rather than sensory attributes but it has value in deciding acceptable standards (e.g., public water supply). Multidimensional scaling uses paired stimuli that are compared for their similarity or differences on a rating scale. The process is repeated for several attributes such as intensity or pleasantness and from this a model is generated for each odor. Allowance is made for individual response differences and overall multidimensional scaling seems to be more robust for scientific work.

Some have proposed that smells are appreciated as a whole and that this in some way hinders analysis. It is suggested that the characterization of odor is more like describing a human face than describing a scene. To communicate facial appearances the easiest method is to point out resemblances to other faces rather than to describe the shape of the nose or eyes. Similarly, odors are perhaps best described by reference to other smells rather than by their primary qualities. Professionals but not amateurs are capable of recognizing the ingredients of several components in a mixture. This requires knowledge of the smells of each compound and how they are changed when mixed together. This is thought to imply that the neural message representing a single odor is not structured differently from that of a complex odor.

If exposure to a novel odor is associated with a significant event, it is stored in long-term memory—apparently after only a single exposure, and with similar reliability to those odors that are deliberately learned. The ability of smell to evoke memories from the distant past is well recognized and exemplified in the writings of Marcel Proust. In a famous passage from his novels *Remembrance of Things Past* (1913), Proust was in the bedroom of his Aunt Leonie when he detected the aroma of petit madeleines (sponge cakes) dipped in tea. This immediately brought forth a vivid memory of an old gray house with a clarity that could not be surpassed by the sight or feel of the madeleine. Emile Zola, the French novelist, noted that the smell of olives would invariably conjure up scenes of Provence where his childhood was spent. Although the ability of a sensory signal to evoke former memories is not unique to the olfactory system, perhaps the vividness of past recall is distinctive. Vietnam War veterans may suffer severe flashbacks if exposed to the smell of tent mold, jet fuel, or burning flesh. A possible reason for these observations is the strong anatomical connections between the olfactory pathways and the limbic system that is concerned with memory and emotion (see Figure 1-6D). Hence memory, emotion, and smell are frequently seen to be interrelated. This aspect is further exemplified in the novel *Perfume* by Patrick Süskind in which a perfumer incensed [*sic*] by the smell of a young lady was able to track her down by following her body odor. It seems that her odor provoked feelings of extreme violence that culminated in her brutal murder. Conversely, the aromatherapist attempts to relax individuals by massage or bathing with odors thought to be soothing such as lavender or jasmine. Use of the steroid musk "Osmone 1" is claimed to have tranquilizing effects and has been proposed as a benzodiazepine substitute.

In military circles there has been rekindling of interest at the prospect of using odor to produce feelings of panic and widespread disarray in wartime. An early contender that smelled of stale garbage was known as "Who Me?," but when it was released it tended to blow back in the face of the assailants! Hydrogen sulphide gas (bad eggs) causes powerful activation of the amygdala producing feelings of disgust or fear; hence most odors proposed for military use contain this vapor. One of the Pentagon's most repugnant smells, "U.S. Government Standard Bathroom Malodor," causes volunteers to scream and curse within a few seconds' exposure. Cultural differences, mentioned later in this chapter, have made it difficult to create a cross-racially repugnant smell and at present the ideal stink bomb has yet to be devised.

ODOR MEMORY IN THE ELDERLY

Healthy elderly persons have a diminished capacity to identify, discriminate, and remember odors. It is well recognized that with advancing years the ability to identify smells declines (Figure 1-12). Doty

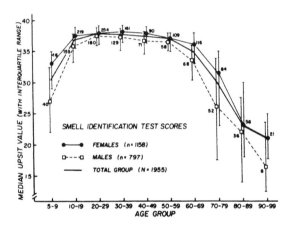

Figure 1-12. Scores on the University of Pennsylvania Smell Identification test as a function of age and gender. Numbers by data points indicate sample sizes. (Reprinted with permission from Doty RL, Shaman P, et al. Smell identification ability: changes with age. Science 1984;226:1441–1443.)

and colleagues, who invented the UPSIT (see Figure 1-12), showed that scores dwindle for both sexes after the age of 70 years. The decrement is quite steep thereafter such that a healthy 90-year-old will identify correctly only half the odors identified by a 20-year-old. Contrary to expectation, UPSIT score does not correlate with memory score as measured on the Wechsler Memory Scale.

In one interesting experiment by Engen and coworkers elderly subjects were asked to identify odors at intervals varying from 0–30 seconds. When there was no delay, 80% of the odors were identified accurately, but if the delay was increased to 30 seconds the accuracy of recognition declined to only 56%. Young volunteers easily outperformed the elderly group. Further experiments suggest that this decline of smell sense with age is not paralleled by a similar deterioration in visual memory.

It is probable that impairment in one aspect of memory such as verbal or visual will materially influence another such as olfaction. A healthy young person probably uses "verbal labeling" to provide a meaningful association to a specific odor. An elderly person may identify a substance as "fruity" but fail to perceive it as apple-like because of the age-related impairment of verbal association memories.

DEMOGRAPHY

In 1986 a massive worldwide analysis of olfaction was undertaken by Wysocki and colleagues through the readership of the *National Geographic* magazine. Nearly 11 million subscribers were asked about basic demography, subjective ability to smell, use of perfume, ability to smell, and subjective rating of androstenone (urinous), amyl-acetate (banana-like), galaxolide (musky), eugenol (cloves), mercaptans (sulphurous, often added to natural gas), and rose scents. On the basis of approximately 1.42 million replies a wealth of data was obtained. Women from the United States scored highest in their self-rating of smell sense and this aspect applied generally to females in the rest of the world. Males from Europe gave themselves the lowest ratings. With respect to the 6 test odors mentioned, all except androstenone and mercaptans were in general rated pleasant irrespective of nationality and gender. Males rated amyl-acetate, androstenone, and mercaptans more pleasant than did females whereas females rated galaxolide, eugenol, and rose more pleasant than did males. Androstenone, a gonadal steroid, is perceived (if at all) either as stale urine, musk-like, or sweet. People who rated androstenone as unpleasant generally gave this a high intensity rating—especially participants from Europe. This observation correlates with other data suggesting that if a subject has a low threshold to the perception of androstenone it is rated unpleasant; if the threshold is high then it will be rated indifferent or pleasant. Amyl-acetate was given a fairly uniform hedonic rating whereas for galaxolide there were major differences. It received lowest pleasantness rating in Asian individuals and highest in Australians, 50% of whom said they would be prepared to wear it as perfume. Although the majority thought that mercaptans were unpleasant there was one exception: those from India liked it! About 70% of Asians were not willing to eat something that smelled like eugenol whereas 30% of whites were prepared to do so. Many other regional differences were noted and this presumably reflects cultural and other environmental differences. One reason for hedonic responses to different odors was suggested to depend on the degree of physical contact between friends and relatives—North European countries being mainly "noncontact" cultures while those from Southern Europe are primarily "contact" societies. Four of the six odors evoked a vivid memory and this was true throughout the world. Galaxolide and to a lesser degree mercaptans were the two least likely to evoke graphic memories. The ability to identify the six odors was fairly uniform worldwide.

Androstenone gave most difficulty with only 20% responding correctly. Galaxolide was just as difficult, especially for men. This information concurs with the well-recognized specific anosmia to either androstenone or galaxolide. Androstenone anosmia was present in 33% of males and 24% of females from America in contrast to 22% of males and 14% of females from Africa. Note that these estimates are slightly lower than those of Wysocki and Beauchamp (see Table 1-1).

In summary, age, and to lesser degree, gender, and smoking habit influence smell identification and perception skills. Odor memory is a major determinant of smell perception. Examination of olfactory experience is severely limited by lack of vocabulary. Although it shares long- and short-term characteristics with verbal memory, for example, odor memory may be represented as a whole. The strong anatomical connections with learning and emotional centers in the temporal lobes may explain the ability of aromas to jog memory vividly. With advancing years odor identification ability and memory decline steeply. The ability to name and detect odors varies widely according to race and sex; pleasantness ratings depend strikingly on social or racial attributes.

Exposure to environmental toxins, drug use and abuse, and a variety of diseases will be discussed in Chapter 3.

SUGGESTED READING

Amoore JE. Specific anosmia: a clue to the olfactory code. Nature 1967 Jun 10;214:1095–1098.

Engen T, Kuisma JE, Eimas PD. Short-term memory of odors. J Exp Psychol 1973;99:222–225.

Frye RE, Schwartz BS, Doty RL. Dose-related effects of cigarette smoking on olfactory function. JAMA 1990 Mar 2;263:1233–1236.

Kobal G, Van Toller S, Hummel T. Is there directional smelling? Experientia 1989;45:130–132.

Pain S. Can you imagine the most terrifying smell in the world? New Scientist 2001 July:43–45.

Proust M. Remembrance of Things Past. Translated by CK Scott-Moncrieff and T Kilmartin. New York: Alfred A. Knopf, 1982.

Sobel N, Prabhakaran V, Hartley CA, et al. Blind smell: brain activation induced by an undetected airborne chemical. Brain 1999;122:209–217.

Süskind, P. Perfume, The Story of a Murderer. Translated from the German by John E. Woods. New York: Alfred A. Knopf, 1986.

Wysocki CJ, Beauchamp GK. Individual differences in human olfaction. In CJ Wysocki, MR Kare (eds), Chemical Senses, Volume 3. Genetics of Perception and Communication. New York: Marcel Dekker Inc., 1991;353–373.

Wysocki CJ, Gilbert AN. National Geographic smell survey. Effects of age are heterogenous. Ann N Y Acad Sci 1989;561:12–28.

Zozulya S, Echeverri F, Nguyen T. The human olfactory receptor repertoire. Genome Biol 2001;2(6): 0018.1–0018.12.

Clinical Methods of Evaluation of Smell

Certain terms need definition and are summarized in Table 2-1. *Anosmia* means absence of smell sense; *hyposmia* or *microsmia* is reduction of it; *dysosmia* means distortion of smell and is divided into *parosmia* (rarely termed *troposmia*) in which the distortion is in response to a specific stimulus and *phantosmia* in which no external stimulus is present. *Cacosmia* is a form of dysosmia where the distortion is—as is often the case—unpleasant. The term *torquosmia* is a rarely used term referring to a smell distortion akin to burning. *Hyperosmia* refers to hypersensitivity to common odors. *Osmophobia* is dislike of certain smells and *presbyosmia* is the natural decline in smell sense with age. Henkin

Table 2-1. Definition of various terms used to describe smell disorder

Term	Definition
Anosmia	Absence of smell sense
Hyposmia or microsmia	Reduction of smell sense
Dysosmia	Distortion of smell sense
Parosmia or troposmia	Distortion due to a specific stimulus
Phantosmia	Distortion when there is no external stimulus
Cacosmia	Unpleasant type of distortion
Torquosmia	Burning type of distortion
Hyperosomia	Increased sensitivity to common odor
Osmophobia	Dislike of certain smells
Heterosmia	All odors smell the same
Presbyosmia	Decline of smell sense with age
Type 1 hyposmia	Inability to recognize stimulus with varying degrees of detection
Type 2 hyposmia	Decreased detection or recognition
Type 3 hyposmia	Reduced intensity ability with normal detection and recognition

divides smell (and taste) impairment into three categories: type 1 is absence of stimulus recognition with varying degrees of smell detection, type 2 is decreased ability to detect or recognize stimuli, and type 3 is decreased ability to judge stimulus intensity with normal detection and recognition thresholds. In *heterosmia* all odors smell the same, although *homosmia* would be a better term.

HISTORY AND EXAMINATION

Patients may not recognize there is a problem with smell unless this faculty is essential for their work or hobbies (e.g., a chef or wine taster). Hence patients must be questioned specifically about it (Tables 2-2 and 2-3). Even when asked, a significant percentage of patients will be unaware of impairment especially in the following circumstances:

- If there is cognitive impairment.
- If the defect is unilateral.
- If the anosmia is long-standing.
- If it came on gradually.

When anosmia is present the patient often confuses it with taste, stating that food tastes bland but only rarely are the two modalities impaired in tandem. The history should be directed particularly to

Table 2-2. Checklist of questions for patient with smell symptoms

Is there loss of taste as well as smell?

Was smell sense normal previously?

Duration of smell loss.

Is it intermittent, continual, or seasonal?

If intermittent is it related to breathing in or out?

Was permanent smell loss of sudden or gradual onset, bilateral or unilateral?

Effect of food? Does food mask a phantom smell?

Can patient smell anything at all and if so what?

Was there a preceding event such as viral infection or trauma?

Are smells perceived without a stimulus (phantosmia) or distorted after stimulus (parosmia) and what is the abnormal smell like?

Is there a history of nose bleeds, facial numbness, visual problems, tearing, overlying skin change?

Is there history of chronic rhinosinusitis, or surgery to nose?

Are there symptoms of unilateral nasal obstruction?

Past medical history. Drug history. Systems review

Social and occupational history. Any possibility of smell impairment from work exposure.

Smoker or non-smoker?

Modified with permission from Cullen MM, Leopold DA. Disorders of smell and taste. Med Clin North Am 1999;83:57–74.

Table 2-3. Main areas of physical examination in anosmic patient

Region	Main Observation or Test
Ears	Serous otitis media including naso-pharyngeal mass or inflammation
Nose	Anterior rhinoscopy for nasal mass, clot, polyps, inflammation of nasal membrane, appearance of nasal skin and bones. Mucosal biopsy if granulomatous or malignant disease suspected.
Eyes	Hypertelorism, tearing
Oral cavity	Nasopharyngeal mass
Neck	Palpate for masses or thyroid enlargement
Suspected neurological problem	Cranial nerves, cerebellum, limb function
Suspected psychiatric problem	Nasal foreign bodies

Modified with permission from Cullen MM, Leopold DA. Disorders of smell and taste. Med Clin North Am 1999;83:57–74.

exclude local nasal or sinus disease. It is helpful to know the time of onset of the smell problem and whether it dated to any causative agent described in more detail in the next chapter such as upper respiratory tract infection, nasal or sinus disease, head/nasal/neck trauma, work in dusty environment, or nasal or sinus surgery. Smoking habit needs to be documented. A drug history may be revealing (qv) and many systemic diseases such as diabetes or renal disease can be relevant.

Smell impairment, like deafness, can be categorized into conductive and sensorineural types. Before any assessment of smell ability can be made it is essential to determine whether the inhaled air can reach the olfactory receptors in the nose. If smell loss arises because air is unable to reach the olfactory epithelium it is conductive. As mentioned earlier, because of the physiological nasal cycle in most people, only one nostril is open at a time. One should be alert to patients who mouth-breathe as they most likely have local disease that could affect their ability to smell. If the patient has a cold, hay fever, or migraine attack, all of which are associated with nasal congestion, then no reliable assessment can be made. Patients with local nasal congestion or obstruction may be asymptomatic but a clue is that hyposmia if it fluctuates is likely to be conductive in origin as it will reflect the degree of nasal congestion. Certain activities reduce congestion (exercise, heavy lifting, or showering) and this variability can aid diagnosis. Simple inspection with a pair of nasal forceps may reveal the patency of the nasal airway peripherally and whether there is obstruction from congestion, polyps, or deviation of the nasal septum. This method will only detect about 50% of pathologies because the olfactory epithelium is located high in the attic. Nasal endoscopy is the only means of examining the olfactory epithelium and can be extremely helpful in differentiating, for example, congenital and traumatic anosmia from viral anosmia. It is useful for identifying nasal tumors, particularly polyps arising high within the nasal cavity (Color Plates 3A–C).

Ideally, all cranial nerves should be examined in someone with a smell problem. The more essential cranial nerves for evaluation are (1) the optic nerve: an abnormal visual field, pupillary defect, optic disk swelling, or atrophy would infer the presence of a frontal lobe tumor or related structural pathology; and (2) the trigeminal nerve. The sensory component is of particular relevance. Common sensation should be assessed over the face with cotton wool and a pin. Nasal tickle is a less well-known stimulant of pain pathways in the nasal mucosa as it is shared with itching and thermal sensation. It is examined by gently moving a wisp of cotton wool inside one nostril. Normal people respond by flinching rapidly and asymmetry would suggest a disorder of trigeminal fine nerve fibers.

Patients with a frontal lobe lesion may have primitive reflexes such as a pout or grasp reflex. When present, a grasp reflex usually indicates bifrontal disease. Simple tests of cognitive function such as the Minimental test are useful means of detecting Alzheimer's disease, a disorder regularly associated with olfactory impairment. A demented patient with memory problems will have difficulty with smell identification tests, making tests of threshold or simple perception more appropriate. Examination should also include the ears and upper respiratory tract.

Rhinomanometry measures the ability to breathe through the nose by placing a sealed system in the right and left nostril independently and asking the patient to breathe in and out. The volume, rate of airflow, and the pressure required to generate this airflow is measured and expressed as resistance to air flow that in turn corresponds to the degree of nasal obstruction. Rhinomanometry can be performed before and after the application of a decongestant such as ephedrine. This helps to quantify the degree of reversible obstruction. Unfortunately such procedures do not measure reliably the olfactory area flow because most airflow is below this level.

Nasal cytology is a useful diagnostic procedure based on histological examination of nasal mucus. In allergic rhinitis there is an excess of eosinophils and basophils, in infectious disorder there are bacteria and polymorphonuclear white cells, and in neoplastic disorder malignant cells may be detected.

Skin tests are useful in patients with hyposmia secondary to allergic rhinitis. This may help to identify the possible allergen and evaluate the need for desensitization. Elevated blood IgE level is suggestive of allergic disorder.

Ciliary motility test. In healthy individuals there is a continual process of transporting trapped particles and mucus to the back of the nose by ciliary activity. In chronic inflammatory disease mucociliary clearance is impaired. This can be assessed by placing a small quantity of saccharine, usually with a marker dye, at the entrance to the nose. The saccharine is propelled backwards and after an interval of 15–20 minutes a sweet taste is perceived and the dye can be seen in the pharynx. In motility disorder the time taken is increased, but the test does not have universally agreed standards.

Identification and threshold tests. Simple olfactory testing is rendered particularly difficult because of the mixed nerve supply of the nose (i.e., olfactory and trigeminal nerves). The majority of commonly used test odors causes simultaneous activation of trigeminal and olfactory nerve endings within the nose (especially ammonia, menthol, and camphor). In addition, many ingredients found in test kits are rarely found in everyday life, and will be difficult to identify particularly for males (e.g., camphor, eucalyptus, oil of cloves, oil of wintergreen).

Tinct. Asafetida, apart from being the most readily recalled and unpleasant (fecal) odorant in some conventional kits, is actually quite a selective olfactory stimulant. For a simple basic screening test, vanilla, chocolate, and coffee are good stimulants and may be identified by most; phenylethyl alcohol is obtainable as a liquid and gives a rose-like odor and is worth including. It was shown by Doty many years ago that anosmic patients could detect acetone, pyridine (fishy), toluene (glue smell), methanol, amylacetate (banana), menthol, linalool (soapy), camphor, methyl-ethyl ketone (glue smell), and many more. The mechanism of detection is probably via trigeminal stimulation although the threshold to a given odor is much higher. Hence a smell test-kit that incorporates any of the latter has dubious value unless the concentrations are very carefully defined.

University of Pennsylvania Smell Identification Test (UPSIT). If more detailed analysis is needed one may use the UPSIT. This employs the scratch and sniff principle (i.e., odor is released on scratching an impregnated cardboard strip; Figure 2-1). For each of 40 test smells (in the standard kit), the subject makes a forced choice from 4 alternatives. Normative values are available for about 4000 Americans standardized for age and sex (see Figure 1-12) but outside America it is essential to establish local control scores. In general, healthy peo-

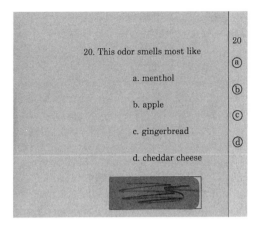

Figure 2-1. A page from the University of Pennsylvania Smell Identification Test. Patients scratch with a pencil the strip on the lower part of the figure, sniff the odor, and make a forced choice from one of four possible answers supplied. Their response is recorded by marking the appropriate letter on the right.

ple under 60 years should score at least 30/40, but anosmics will attain an average of 10 ± 5. Clever malingerers score 0–5 as they intentionally de-select the correct answer and they are likely to scratch the impregnated strip less vigorously than a genuine hyposmic. The UPSIT-40 has proved a reliable procedure and is useful for both routine clinical and medicolegal cases. It has high test–retest reliability and should be regarded as the screening test of choice for clinical and research procedures. It does, however, assess cognitive function at the same time—the more intelligent person may not recognize the correct odor but could identify those that are wrong, and deduce the correct answer by elimination. This drawback offsets its usefulness in Alzheimer's disease, for example, where smell memory, concentration, and reasoning may be affected and tests of perception or threshold would be more appropriate. Non-Americans may have difficulty with some of the forced choices (e.g., skunk, pumpkin pie, root beer). To avoid this problem there is an international version that has just 12 odorants. Although this is good for basic clinical screening it is not suitable for research purposes as it provides insufficient statistical precision. For those with a time problem there is a pocket smell test with just 3 common odors. Anything is better than sticky bottles containing oil of cloves, camphor, peppermint, and so on.

A rival assessment uses "sniffin' sticks." This procedure consists of a collection of felt-tip pens impregnated with various smells. Published normative data are available for over 1,000 German people (Kobal et al., 2000) and may be expressed as a threshold, discrimination, and identification score (TDI index). Despite this it is essential to establish local population control data if any research investigation is contemplated. Sniffin' sticks will be more time consuming to use if the TDI score is required but in the long run they are considerably cheaper after the initial outlay. Contact information for suppliers of these products is supplied in the appendix.

A more refined approach is to determine the absolute level of a particular odorant that can be detected. Air-dilution olfactometry would be the method of choice but this requires complex apparatus and is not practical for ordinary clinical investigation. A good compromise is to use an odorant such as phenylethyl-alcohol (rose smelling) in varying dilutions contained in small flasks held under the nose (sniff bottles). Using serial dilutions on an ascending log scale, a fairly accurate measure of olfactory threshold to one particular odor may be obtained. Somewhat similar is the "T & T olfactometer" or perfumists' strip (Figure 2-2). This consists of 8 $\log_{10}$ serial dilutions of 5 odorants: phenylethylalcohol (rose-like), methyl-cyclopentenolene (fruity), isovaleric acid (sweaty), gamma undecalactone (caramel), and skatole (fecal). The samples are taken on a piece of filter paper and held under the nose. Threshold tests are less influenced by cognitive function and, theoretically at least, should be better than identification procedures.

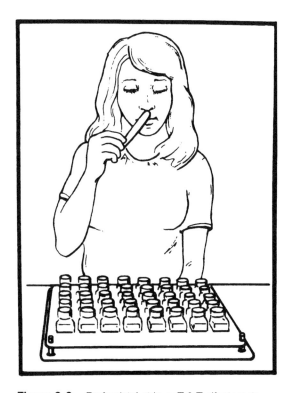

Figure 2-2. Perfumists' strip or T & T olfactometer. (Reprinted with permission from Doty R, Kobal G. Current trends in the measurement of olfactory function. In RL Doty (ed), Handbook of Olfaction and Gustation. New York: Marcel Dekker Inc., 1995; Chapter 8.)

Threshold tests correlate well with the UPSIT but they take much longer to perform so most people prefer identification tests as long as cognitive function is normal.

There is no specific test for dysosmia although the majority of patients with this complaint have some degree of olfactory loss, typically of mild or moderate severity.

Olfactory evoked tests. A difficulty with all the previously discussed tests is that they are subjective and evaluate cognitive function to varying degrees. Olfactory evoked potentials (OEP) or some would prefer the term chemosensory evoked responses, represent one of the more sophisticated and objective tests and were pioneered by Kobal and Plattig (1978). Selected odors are embedded in a fast-flowing airstream that enters the nostril by way of a short piece of Teflon tubing, thus avoiding trigeminal stimulation (Figure 2-3 and Color Plate 4). By introducing a short odor pulse (i.e., 200 milliseconds) an evoked potential is obtained from the vertex after an interval of approximately 400 milliseconds or more. It is objective and less dependent on cognitive factors and this, in principle, makes it more valuable than the UPSIT and threshold tests. It is a useful way (and perhaps the only reliable method) of detecting malingerers. Data for disease states such as multiple sclerosis and Parkinson's disease (Figure 2-4) are

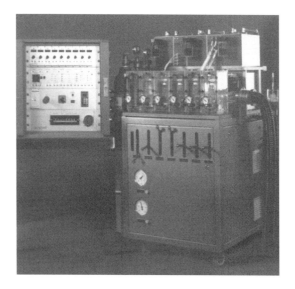

Figure 2-3. A commercially available four-odorant olfactometer (Burghart OM4).

now available. Because of the complexity and expense of apparatus, OEP is still a research procedure.

Plain radiographs have substantial limitations; they do not provide sufficient detail for structures such as the osteomeatal complex. In particular, more detailed images are needed when endoscopic surgery is to be performed. Computed tomographic

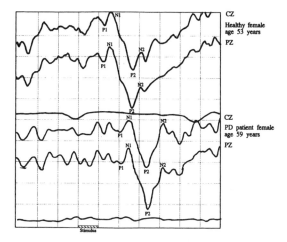

Figure 2-4. Sample of olfactory evoked response in normal person. Upper pair of traces is derived from CZ and PZ in a healthy female aged 53 years. The third tracing is an eye artifact monitor. The next pair of tracings is from a 59-year-old patient with idiopathic Parkinson's disease. There is clear delay of responses at CZ and PZ. Note the slightly larger response from PZ in both cases. Bottom trace is again the eye movement channel. The stimulant was a 200mS pulse of H_2S at a concentration of 20ppm in both cases. Filters are set at 1–50Hz. Squares represent 6.25µV on vertical axis and 200mS on horizontal axis.

(CT) scanning is the most useful and cost-effective technique for evaluating sinonasal tract inflammatory disorders. Coronal CT scans are particularly valuable in assessing paranasal anatomy. Scanning with thin cuts (5 mm) identifies bony structures in the ethmoid, cribriform plate, and olfactory cleft, as well as the temporal bone in proximity to cranial nerve VII or chorda tympani nerves. CT used with intravenous contrast media is better at identifying vascular lesions, tumors, abscess cavities, and meningeal or parameningeal processes. However, CT scanning is less effective than magnetic resonance imaging (MRI) in defining soft tissue disease. MRI is superior to CT scanning in the evaluation of soft tissues, but it defines bony structures poorly and tends to overemphasize mucosal disease. MRI is the technique of choice for assessing the olfactory bulbs, olfactory tracts, facial nerve, and intracranial causes of chemosensory dysfunction. It is also the preferred technique for evaluating the skull base for invasion by sinonasal tumors. Gadolinium enhancement helps to detect dural or leptomeningeal involvement at the skull base.

Brain mapping is an alternative method of image enhancement that allows spatial distribution of the electroencephalogram (EEG) to be displayed in the form of a contour map. The result is aesthetically pleasing and allows the distribution of brain activity to be visualized more readily than does simple inspection of the EEG. When used with evoked potential studies it has shown that pure olfactory signals such as vanillin are maximally represented in the central parietal zones (PZ) whereas impure odors (i.e., those with trigeminal activity) such as ammonia cause a response slightly more anteriorly at CZ, implying a different generator site.

Functional magnetic resonance imaging (fMRI) and positron emission tomography (PET) are the most sophisticated measurements of cerebral activity in response to odor. Initial studies have confirmed that the main olfactory association area is in the right orbitofrontal cortex (see Color Plate 4). Disease-related functional olfactory studies are just beginning and both of these techniques at present belong to the domain of research.

Examination of living olfactory neurones. A recent development in olfactory measurement also involves the extraction of living human olfactory cells from the middle turbinate or attic at the time of nasal surgery or as an elective procedure (Figure 2-5). This allows morphological and pharmacological properties of such cells to be examined by, for example, immunoreactive markers and patch clamp studies. Such olfactory neurons can be grown in vitro, albeit with difficulty. These studies have the potential to further our knowledge of

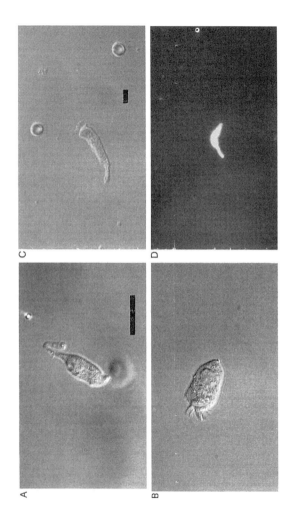

68

Figure 2-5. Sample of cells taken from middle turbinate biopsy sample. **A**, Olfactory receptor neuron. **B**, Respiratory epithelial cell. **C**, Supporting cell. **D**, Olfactory marker protein-positive receptor neuron. Anti-OMP serum, fluorescein isothiocyanate. Scale bar 10μm. (Reprinted with permission from Thuerauf N, Gjuric M, Kobal G, Hatt H. Clinical nucleotide-gated channels in identified human olfactory receptor neurons. European J Neuroscience 1996;8:2080–2089.)

degenerative disease such as Alzheimer's disease and Parkinson's disease in which the olfactory system is known to be involved.

In summary, evaluation of smell sense should commence with a thorough history and clinical examination. This may be supplemented by special tests such as rhinomanometry, cytology, skin, or motility tests as appropriate. Measurement of olfactory function is complex but a reasonable assessment may be attained by UPSIT, sniffin' sticks, or threshold tests. None is completely objective and to avoid bias, evoked potential or brain mapping procedures may be required. So far, olfactory analysis has not achieved the level of sophistication achieved in the visual or auditory sphere.

SUGGESTED READING

Amoore JE. Specific anosmia: a clue to the olfactory code. Nature 1967;214:1095–1098.

Cullen MM, Leopold DA. Disorders of smell and taste. Med Clin North Am 1999;83:57–74.

Doty RL, Shaman P, Kimmelman CP, Dann MS. University of Pennsylvania Smell Identification Test: a rapid quantitative olfactory function test for the clinic. Laryngoscope 1984;94:176–178.

Frye RE, Schwartz BS, Doty RL. Dose-related effects of cigarette smoking on olfactory function. JAMA 1990;263:1233–1236.

Hawkes CH, Shephard BC. Olfactory evoked responses and identification tests in neurological disease. Ann N Y Acad Sci 1998;855:608–615.

Kettenmann B, Francis S, Aspen J, et al. Repeated trigeminal stimuli result in a constant or even sensitized SII activity while olfactory related activity generally shows attenuation. Chem Sens 2001; 26(8):1085–1086.

Kobal G, Hummel C. Cerebral chemosensory evoked potentials elicited by chemical stimulation of the human olfactory and respiratory nasal mucosa. Electroenceph Clin Neurophysiol 1988;71:241–250.

Kobal G, Klimek L, Wolfensberger M, et al. Multicenter investigation of 1,036 subjects using a standardized method for the assessment of olfactory function combining tests of odor identification, odor discrimination, and olfactory thresholds. Eur Arch Otorhinolaryngol 2000;257:205–211.

Kobal G, Plattig KH. Objective olfactometry: methodological annotations for recording olfactory EEG-responses from the awake human. EEG EMG Z Elektroenzephalogr Elektromyogr Verwandte Geb 1978;9:135–145.

Thurauf N, Gjuric M, Kobal G, Hatt H. Cyclic nucleotide-gated channels in identified human olfactory receptor neurons. Eur J Neurosci.1996;8:2080–2089.

Van Toller S, Reed MK. Brain electrical activity topographical maps produced in response to olfactory and chemosensory stimulation. Psychiatry Res 1989;29:429–430.

Wysocki CJ, Gilbert AN. National Geographic Smell Survey. Effects of age are heterogenous. Ann N Y Acad Sci 1989;561:12–28.

Disorders of Olfaction

DISORDERS OF OLFACTORY PERCEPTION

Distortion or perversion in the perception of an odor is known as *parosmia* (rarely known as *troposmia*). If the sensation is unpleasant (as it usually is), the phenomenon is called *cacosmia*. Such perversions are common when there is local nasal disease—typically infection in the sinuses or nose itself—but may be found when there is trauma to the olfactory nerve or bulb following head injury or chemical exposure. Parosmia may be associated with normal or diminished smell sensitivity. Minor degrees of parosmia are not necessarily abnormal—for example, unpleasant smells can linger for several hours and may be subsequently rekindled by other olfactory stimuli.

Hyperosmia

Hyperosmia is a disorder of perception in which there are varying degrees of increased sensitivity to one or more aromas. It has been observed in Addison's disease (adrenal-cortical insufficiency), some cases of head injury, and may follow abrupt drug withdrawal. A minority doubt the existence of the condition in association with physical disease. Certainly some neurotic individuals complain of undue sensitivity to odors when there is no proof of actual change in odor perception threshold. Conversely, it has been shown by smell perception tests that about 2% of healthy individuals are hyperosmic to pyridine. During or before migraine attacks some report temporary heightened and unpleasant smell perception (osmophobia) in a manner comparable to photophobia and phonophobia. Many patients are initially depressed but if not they soon become so. It can form part of a more generalized syndrome of multiple chemical hypersensitivity (MCS) in which numerous symptoms are connected with repeated exposure to environmental chemicals. When Doty and colleagues tested 18 MCS patients for hypersensitivity to two odors there was no difference in olfactory detection threshold but there was a high level of depression, increased nasal resistance to odors, and disordered respiratory rate. This suggested there was a complex mixture of physical, psychiatric, and autonomic problems.

Hallucinations

An olfactory hallucination is a disorder of smell perception in the absence of odor in the environment. The subject claims to smell an odor that no one else can. If the patient is convinced of its presence and also gives it personal reference despite all evidence to the contrary, it is then a delusion and termed *olfactory reference syndrome*, described in the following paragraphs. Olfactory hallucinations may result from disorder almost anywhere along the smell pathway from the nose to the primary olfactory cortex in the medial aspect of the temporal lobes. The orbitofrontal cortex is an association area and probably does not cause hallucinations if diseased. Patients with local nasal problems such as infection or trauma may complain of a continuous or intermittent unpleasant smell (phantosmia) in the absence of any external stimulus.

One of the earliest descriptions of olfactory hallucination was by the famous English neurologist Hughlings Jackson in an account of a cook who experienced epileptic attacks emanating from the temporal lobe: "In the paroxysm the first thing was tremor of the hands and arms; she saw a little black woman who was always very actively engaged in cooking; the spectre did not speak. The patient had a very horrible smell (so-called subjective sensation of smell) that she could not describe. She had a feeling as if she was shut up in a box with a limited quantity of air…she would stand with her eyes fixed … and then say 'what a horrible smell!'… After leaving her kitchen work she had paroxysms with the smell sensation but no spectre." At autopsy there was a large tumor occupying the anterior portion of the temporal lobe. Clearly this growth was irritating the uncus (anteromedially placed in the temporal lobe) and causing the now well-recognized variety of seizure—uncinate epilepsy. In most instances the hallucination is unpleasant and difficult to remember or describe in any more detail, but why this should be is unclear. Conceivably it relates to a simultaneous disturbance in the hippocampal formation that is known to be concerned with short-term memory.

Apart from uncinate seizures, olfactory hallucinations and delusions usually signify a psychiatric illness. There is complaint of a large variety of smells, mainly foul. A patient may mistakenly believe that a foul smell emanates from himself (intrinsic hallucination) and may be attributing this to something wrong with the nose. In others the odors seem to come from an external source (extrinsic hallucination). In a review of depressed patients Pryse-Phillips found olfactory symptoms to be an early and predominating complaint in half of his patients with typical endogenous depression and termed this *olfactory reference syndrome*. They usually suffered from intrinsic hallucinations whereas those due to schizophrenia had extrinsic hallucinations apparently induced by someone for the purpose of upsetting the patient. Reactions to the hallucinations varied from none at all to petitioning police and neighbors or continual washing and social withdrawal.

Stereotactic lesions of the amygdala can abolish both olfactory hallucinations and the accompanying psychiatric disorder, which would imply that the amygdaloid nuclei are the source of hallucinatory activity. Olfactory hallucinations and delusions are seen in senile dementia sometimes in the absence of depression. They are also associated with alcohol withdrawal.

Agnosia

Failure to recognize or identify aromas in the presence of normal ability to discriminate differences between them would be termed olfactory agnosia.

Extremely few cases of this have been described, which is surprising in view of the well-recognized forms of agnosia in the visual and auditory spheres. It has been associated with right inferior temporal lesions in association with agnosia for familiar faces (prosopagnosia).

Effect of Drugs

Many drugs are claimed to interfere with smell sense (Table 3-1). It should be emphasized that several reports relate to single examples and often no formal smell or taste examination has been undertaken—the patient's account is relied on. Considering how many patients (and clinicians) confuse the two modalities, the alleged associations should be viewed with circumspection. It must also be considered that the disease for which a drug is given (e.g., diabetes or thyroid disorder) may be the cause of smell dysfunction and not the drug itself. Drugs thought to affect smell sense include calcium channel blockers, antibiotics, antithyroid drugs, opiates, antidepressants, and sympathomimetics. Many lipid-lowering drugs give rise to hyposmia and they are thought to act by decreasing tissue levels of vitamin A that is concerned with olfactory receptor function. Sudden withdrawal of benzodiazepines or antidepressants may produce hyperosmia. The most convincing evidence for drug-induced olfactory disturbance comes

Table 3-1. Drugs reported to interfere with smell sense with some examples

Drug Group	Example
Calcium channel blocker	Nifedipine; amlodipine; diltiazem
Lipid lowering	Cholestyramine; clofibrate; pravastatin
Antibiotic and antifungal	Streptomycin; doxycycline; terbinafine
Antithyroid	Carbimazole
Opiate	Codeine; morphine
Antidepressant	Amitriptyline
Sympathomimetic	Dexamphetamine; phenmetrazine
Antiepileptic	Phenytoin
Nasal decongestant	Phenylephrine; pseudoephedrine; oxymetazoline (long-term use probably required for damage)
Miscellaneous	Smoking, argyria (topical application of silver nitrate), cadmium fumes; phenothiazines; pesticides; Betnesol-N; cocaine (snorted)
Organic solvents	See Table 3-3

from accounts of inhaled organic chemicals. This would be expected because they have direct access to the olfactory epithelium. Likewise snorted recreational drugs such as cocaine are sometimes associated with anosmia because of destruction to the olfactory epithelium or nasal septum. It is probable that the risk for smell loss in this group has been overstated and permanent smell loss is unusual. Nasal decongestants are an occasional cause of hyposmia and in some cases the defect is persistent.

DISEASE AFFECTING OLFACTION

It is difficult to classify olfactory disease (Table 3-2). About 50% of those presenting to rhinology clinics will have conductive loss. Once this type of loss is eliminated, lesions of the first cranial nerve, which takes a long course and may involve damage at multiple sites (sometimes simultaneously), must be considered. Causes will be arbitrarily divided into peripheral and central causes, although it is inevitable that there will be some overlap. Relative proportions of the various causes are shown in the pie chart in Figure 3-1.

PERIPHERAL CAUSES

Local Nasal Disease

This is the most common reason for anosmia and is called *conductive* when air is prevented from reaching the olfactory receptors. Any obstructive or inflammatory process can be responsible, such as hay

Table 3-2. List of main categories of disease causing smell disturbance with typical examples*

Disease Category	Example
Local nasal	Polyps, hay fever, sinus disease
Endocrinopathy	Diabetes; Addison's, Cushing's, and Klinefelter's syndromes; pseudohypo-parathyroidism; Kallmann's syndrome; septo-optic dysplasia
Viral and infectious	Common cold, influenza, herpes encephalitis, AIDS, prion disease
Head injury	Usually severe posterior or lateral impact
Epilepsy	Olfactory aura, complex partial seizure
Migraine	Before, during, or after attack
Multiple sclerosis	During relapse or in more advanced disease
Tumors and inflammatory disease	Nasopharyngeal carcinoma, Wegener's granulomatosis, olfactory groove meningioma or neuroblastoma, facial Paget's disease, Sjögren's syndrome
Neurodegenerative disease	See Table 3-4

*Neurodegenerative causes are listed in Table 3-4.

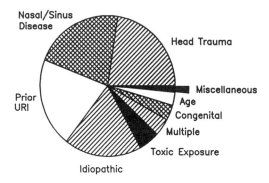

Figure 3-1. Proportion of patients in various diagnostic categories of olfactory impairment among 200 patients at University of Cincinnati Taste and Smell Center. Four categories (nasal/sinus disease, head injury, upper respiratory infection, and idiopathic) account for 83% of all patients. (Reprinted with permission from Duncan HJ, Smith DV. Clinical disorders of olfaction. In RL Doty (ed), Handbook of Olfaction and Gustation. New York: Marcel Dekker Inc., 1995; Chapter 14.)

fever, polyps (particularly in the vault), inflammatory disease of the ethmoid or maxillary sinuses, osteomeatal disease, deformity due to trauma, malignant disease of the nose, paranasal sinuses, or nasopharynx. If there is chronic nasal sinus disease the mucus clearance rate is reduced because of disordered ciliary motility. This along with inflammation contributes to hyposmia. Recent studies indicate that in as many as 70% of those with olfactory disturbance, the nasal airway may remain patent despite obstruction of the nasal vault. Oddly enough, mild or moderate congestion of the turbinates in the absence of disease does not necessarily cause impairment of smell function and may actually enhance it, perhaps by providing extra humidity and some resistance to airflow. Likewise the cyclical diurnal variation of nasal resistance on one side does not cause hyposmia. Nasal dryness, which occurs where there has been excessive surgery, atrophic rhinitis, or Sjögren's syndrome, will cause anosmia as a moist olfactory receptor area is essential for smell perception.

Viral and Infectious Illness

This is the most frequent cause of anosmia. Even the common cold may damage olfaction temporarily or permanently. Hepatitis, flu-like infections, herpes simplex encephalitis, and most recently variant Creutzfeldt-Jakob disease are rare causes of olfactory dysfunction and presumably relate to direct viral attack on the olfactory pathways, either peripherally in the nasal olfactory epithelium or olfactory bulb, or centrally in the temporal lobes. Usually smell loss is not complete but in contrast to conductive anosmia the symptoms are stable. Patients with the more common forms of post-viral hyposmia tend to be older, female, and complain of dysosmia. Most patients in this category gradually improve but over a prolonged period of up to 5 years.

Toxic Anosmia

There are numerous compounds alleged to cause anosmia; the majority occurs at work and inevitably promotes lawsuits. The main compounds that cause acute olfactory loss with variable degrees of recovery are listed in Table 3-3. Many instances are single case reports and usually patients' symptomatic reports have been relied on in the absence of formal olfactory testing. More substantive evidence is available for the following metallic compounds causing permanent hyposmia following chronic exposure (either as base metal or salt): chrome, lead, mercury, nickel, silver, steel, zinc, cadmium. Dust exposure is also related to permanent smell loss following chronic exposure (e.g., cement, hardwood, lime, printing, and silica). Non-metallic inorganic compounds such as carbon disulphide, carbon monoxide, chlorine, hydrazine, nitrogen dioxide, ammonia, sulphur dioxide, and fluorides on chronic exposure have been linked to permanent hyposmia. Organic compounds that also produce permanent hyposmia following chronic exposure include acetone, acetophenone, benzine, chloromethane, menthol, pentachlorophenol, and trichloroethylene. Certain manufacturing processes

Table 3-3. List of substances associated with temporary or permanent toxic hyposmia with varying recovery

Substance	Exposure Period	Symptom
A. Acute exposure with temporary hyposmia		
Formaldehyde	Minutes	Hyposmia
Hydrogen cyanide	Seconds	Anosmia
Hydrogen selenide	Minutes	Hyposmia
Hydrogen sulphide	Seconds	Anosmia
B. Acute exposure, recoverable hyposmia		
Hydrogen selenide	One sniff	Anosmia
N-methylformimino-methylester	One sniff	Anosmia
Sulphuric acid	One sniff	Anosmia
Zinc sulphate	Seconds	Anosmia
C. Acute exposure, permanent hyposmia		
Cesspool	Hours	Anosmia
Decomposing cadaver	Hours	Anosmia
Pepper and cresol powder	One sniff	Hyposmia and cacosmia
Phosphorus oxy-chloride and sulphur dioxide	One sniff	Anosmia

Adapted from Amoore JE. Effects of chemical exposure on olfaction in humans. In CS Barrow (ed), Toxicology of the Nasal Passages. New York; London: McGraw-Hill; 1986:155–190.

are also likely to cause permanent hyposmia after chronic exposure (e.g., manufacture of asphalt, fragrances, lead-based paint, paprika, spices, tobacco, varnishes, waste water refining, and use of cutting oils). It is of interest that painters who smoke experience less impairment of smell sense than nonsmokers, suggesting that smoking is protective against some airborne toxins. There are many anecdotal reports of hyposmia from acute or chronic exposure in the workplace and for further information the reader is referred to the review by Amoore (1986).

Head Injury

There are both peripheral and central causes of smell disturbance related to head injury but the peripheral variety is far more common. The various sites of damage are shown in Figure 3-2. In the primarily neurological sphere, head injury is the most common cause of anosmia and is usually attributed to shearing of olfactory nerve fibers as they emerge from the cribriform plate to enter the bulb above it. To produce post-traumatic anosmia the skull usually has to be fractured. A gentle blow to the head or even acceleration forces such as whiplash injury may on very rare occasion be sufficient to cause anosmia, a point of considerable relevance to medicolegal work. Anosmia is most likely to happen (according to traditional wisdom) if the

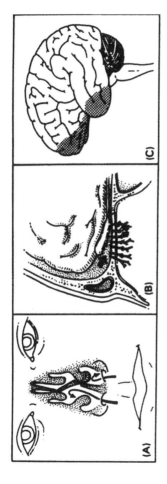

Figure 3-2. Mechanisms of traumatic olfactory dysfunction. **A**, Injury to sinonasal tract. **B**, Tearing of the olfactory nerves. **C**, Cortical contusions and hemorrhage. (Reprinted with permission from Costanzo RM, DiNardo LJ, Zasler ND. Head injury and olfaction. In RL Doty (ed), Handbook of Olfaction and Gustation. New York: Marcel Dekker Inc., 1995; Chapter 21.)

front or back or the head is struck rather than the sides, because it is said that the opportunity for shearing forces on the frontal lobes is greater with antero-posterior injury. Doty and colleagues in a detailed survey of 179 head-injured patients assessed by UPSIT and MRI, found that occipital and side impact caused the most damage and frontal impact the least.

Intracranial hemorrhage per se can result in anosmia and ageusia (taste loss) as well. Lesions that have been associated with post-traumatic anosmia are usually located in the temporal lobes but recent functional imaging studies (SPECT) suggest that the orbitofrontal cortex is hypoperfused, and these patients regularly have other frontal lobe dysfunction. The frequency of traumatic anosmia has been estimated at 7% in head injury of all varieties, rising to 30% when injury is severe and particularly when there is cerebrospinal fluid rhinorrhea. However, many earlier studies, although based on series of over 1000 cases, have used unsophisticated measurement or simply relied on patients' symptoms. Sometimes olfactory assessment has been undertaken within the first few weeks of injury, at a time when local nasal swelling or fracture would result in conductive anosmia and a good prospect of recovery. The percentage who recover from post-traumatic anosmia relates as expected to the duration of post-traumatic amnesia, with those amnesic for over 7 days having the poorest outcome.

In the study of head-injured patients by Doty and co-workers there were 67% with anosmia, 20% with microsmia, and only 13% with normal smell sense—a far higher proportion of abnormality than previously documented. The prevalence of parosmia was found to be about 41% but it decreased to 15% over 8 years. Recovery was equally poor: of 66 patients who could be retested 36% improved slightly, 45% were unchanged, and 18% actually worsened. Only 3 patients recovered from initial anosmia. This is much lower than expected in view of the ability of olfactory neurons to regenerate. One reason for failed recovery may relate to the presence of scar tissue in the cribriform plate, which acts as a barrier to regenerating neurons. Another reason would be the presence of traumatic lesions in the frontal and temporal zones, suggesting centrally based anosmia and less prospect of recovery. Clearly some will have both peripheral and central lesions. Finally, MRI volumetric studies in males with post-traumatic anosmia showed that olfactory bulb volume was reduced. The higher prevalence in males was thought to relate to more severe trauma. The presence of bulb hypovolemia would clearly give objective support to patients' symptoms, especially where there was doubt concerning their authenticity. Although the Doty study paints a fairly gloomy picture, there may be selection bias as all subjects were seen in a specialist referral center. The follow-up rate is also low (66 of 179 originally seen) and this would tend to increase artificially the rate of abnormality (i.e., those who recovered would be less likely to return for assessment). Nonetheless, it is the most elaborate study of post-traumatic anosmia so far and although it probably overstates the magnitude of the problem it concurs well with clinical experience that most patients with complete anosmia lasting more than a few months following head trauma do not get better.

Tumors and Nasal Inflammatory Disease

Smell sense is lost regularly when the nose is involved by tumor, most often the benign polyp. Malignant disease, such as adenocarcinoma, squamous carcinoma, or olfactory neuroblastoma, invade the ethmoid or sphenoid sinuses and produce anosmia. Lymphoma may invade the nasal passages or sinuses and granulomatous disease such as congenital syphilis, sarcoidosis, lupus, and particularly Wegener's granulomatosis are associated with anosmia. Many of the latter produce a characteristic "saddle-nose" deformity.

Endocrine Disease

This is less frequently responsible for anosmia, but depression of smell sense is recognized in Addison's disease, Cushing's syndrome, diabetes, myxedema pseudohypoparathyroidism, and Turner's syndrome. Kallmann's syndrome is an X-linked or autosomal recessive neuronal migration disorder with endocrine deficiency. It is associated with usually complete anosmia due to aplasia of the olfactory bulb in association with hypogonadism. In the related condition of congenital maldevelopment of the optic and septal areas (septo-optical aplasia) there is also anosmia and endocrine deficiency.

CENTRAL CAUSES

Neurodegenerative Disease

Of great interest to the neurologist is the observation that certain diseases associated with neuronal degeneration, such as Alzheimer's, Korsakoff's psychosis, and Parkinson's disease are accompanied by disturbance of olfaction (Figures 2-4 and 3-3). It is suggested that lesions within the olfactory system are some of the first to occur in Alzheimer's disease (AD), and certainly the olfactory pathways are pathologically extensively damaged in this form of dementia.

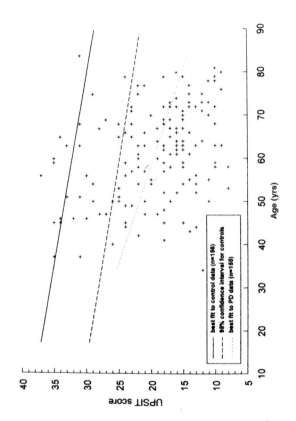

Figure 3-3. UPSIT scores in Parkinson's disease compared to healthy controls. The continuous line is the best fit by age for controls. The long dotted line represents the 95% confidence limit for controls. The fine dotted line is the best fit for Parkinson's disease patients by age. Each + represents the actual UPSIT score for one patient.

The studies of Bacon et al. (1998) imply that elevation of olfactory threshold may be the first change before cognitive impairment ensues. In a prospective population-based study of 1,836 healthy people, Graves et al. (1999) tested smell identification at baseline by the international UPSIT-12 test and a cognitive screening procedure. They found that hyposmia and particularly anosmia significantly increased the risk of subsequent cognitive failure. Anosmics at baseline who had at least one apoliproprotein E-4 (ApoE-4) allele had nearly five times the risk of subsequent cognitive decline. Another group examined prospectively olfactory identification scores in patients with mild cognitive impairment. Those scoring 34 or less on the UPSIT-40, who were also unaware of their defect, were more at risk of developing AD within 2 years.

In Down syndrome (DS) pathological and clinical changes similar to AD develop in adult life. When adult DS patients are compared to other mentally retarded controls the modified UPSIT score is lower. Adolescent DS patients score normally, suggesting that AD pathology develops pari-passu with the olfactory damage, although some argue that because the severity of hyposmia is comparable to older DS patients this implies that smell loss is in fact an early feature.

Patients with the alcoholic form of Korsakoff's psychosis have difficulty in discrimination but no loss of sensitivity. How much of their problem relates to cognitive dysfunction (especially memory) is debated, but the consensus view is that the impairment does not relate to any defect in olfactory acuity, learning ability, or memory. It is likely that the lesion responsible for olfactory discriminatory problems in Korsakoff's psychosis lies in the dorsomedial nucleus of the thalamus, which, as mentioned earlier, has important connections with the orbitofrontal cortex—the main area for olfactory identification and discrimination.

In idiopathic Parkinson's disease (IPD) smell appreciation is impaired at an early stage that anecdotally may predate the motor signs by several years. About 80% of cognitively normal patients with IPD have hyposmia or anosmia as measured by UPSIT-40 or threshold tests but the scores on this test do not deteriorate with time nor do they correlate with disability, depression, or use of anti-parkinsonian drugs. However, olfactory evoked response latency is increased and has been found to correlate with disability. Some have suggested that sniffing is impaired in Parkinson's disease and that this will affect olfactory measurements where sniffing is required. The magnitude of this effect is, however, quite small and the evidence from pathological studies for olfactory damage in IPD is overwhelming. It is not known whether the major olfactory defect is in the olfactory receptor cell, bulb, or more proximally, but pathological change has been shown at all these sites. Such is the frequency of hyposmia in this condition that someone suspected to have IPD with a normal UPSIT-40 score probably has another extrapyramidal disease (see Figure 3-3). It is now established that smokers are less liable to develop PD although their smell identification score may be impaired slightly due to smoking itself. It is speculated that the protective effect of cigarette smoking relates to enhanced cytochrome P450 activity in the nasal mucosa. Some have suggested that PD is a primary disorder of olfaction and the cause relates to an infection or chemical that gains access to the brain through the nose (olfactory vector theory) or that there is a mutation in a gene, perhaps coding for alpha-synuclein, that is expressed in olfactory and extrapyramidal regions.

If indeed smell impairment is the first abnormality in the development of Parkinson's disease then it should be possible to anticipate the development of motor symptoms by olfactory tests. Montgomery and colleagues (1999) administered a test battery to first-degree relatives of IPD patients. The battery included tests of motor function, olfaction, and mood. There were significant differences in first-degree relatives (both sons and daughters) particularly where the affected parent was the father. Another group studied subclinical dopamine dysfunction in asymptomatic IPD patients' relatives who were hyposmic. Single photon emission computed tomography (SPECT) with beta-CIT was used to label the dopamine transporter. Abnormal binding was found in 4 out of 25 hyposmic relatives, 2 of whom subsequently developed IPD. None of the 23 normosmic relatives developed IPD. They suggested that olfactory dysfunction preceded clinical motor signs of the disease. While this may be correct it simply could be easier to detect changes earlier in the olfactory than motor system and a parallel argument could be applied to the early smell changes in AD. Varying degrees of olfactory impairment have been described in other extrapyramidal conditions such as the Guam PD-dementia complex, diffuse Lewy body disease, multiple system atrophy, and drug-induced PD, and these are summarized in Table 3-4.

In schizophrenia there is quite severe olfactory impairment on identification, threshold sensitivity, and odor memory tests. It is of considerable interest that UPSIT scores decline with disease duration in linear fashion, raising the possibility of a disease progression marker.

Table 3-4. Relative degree of olfactory dysfunction in various neurodegenerative conditions on an arbitrary scale

Disease	Severity of Smell Loss
Idiopathic Parkinson's disease	++++
Guam PD-dementia complex	++++
Diffuse Lewy body disease	++++
Familial Parkinson's: affected/ at risk	+++/+
Schizophrenia	+++
Alzheimer's disease	++
Multiple system atrophy	++
Drug-induced PD	++
Down syndrome	+
Huntington's chorea	+
Motor neurone disease	0/+
Progressive supranuclear palsy	0/+
MPTP parkinsonism	0
Cortico-basal degeneration	0
Essential tremor	0
Idiopathic dystonia	0

Key: ++++, marked damage; +, mild; 0, normal. Most of the values are based on relatively small patient numbers except for idiopathic Parkinson's disease.

Epilepsy

The best-known disorder to cause olfactory impairment, albeit transiently, is the uncinate aura. This is an epileptic aura that according to orthodox teaching is caused by irritation of the anteromedial part of the temporal lobe (Figure 3-4). This area, the uncus, is a primary olfactory area (see Figure 1-6). Recent pathological studies suggest that the adjacent amygdala is the site of olfactory aura, so the term "uncinate attack" is possibly a misnomer. The hallucination is usually unpleasant—for example, gas or oil—and may occur in isolation. Sometimes it is followed by a complex partial or secondary generalized tonic-clonic convulsion. It is an ominous symptom that frequently indicates the presence of a malignant tumor. Epilepsy in the frontal lobe does not appear to cause olfactory impairment (although it might theoretically) but if a frontal lobe is removed there is impaired discrimination, which as expected, is bilateral if the right orbitofrontal cortex is ablated. Epilepsy is associated with a generalized decline in olfactory function, but those with complex partial seizures have more impairment than those with generalized epilepsy. Rarely, anticonvulsant therapy such as phenytoin may cause hyposmia (see Table 3-1).

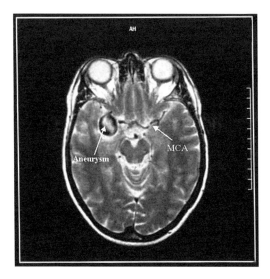

Figure 3-4. T2-weighted axial MRI scan of a large middle cerebral aneurysm involving the antero-medial part of the right temporal lobe (uncus). MCA = middle cerebral artery. This was a 52-year-old woman who complained of unpleasant olfactory hallucinations (uncinate fits), some of which were followed by a generalized tonic-clonic convulsion. Usually uncinate fits are due to a malignant glioma in the temporal lobe.

Migraine

Sufferers of migraine will occasionally report that an attack is provoked by exposure to certain smells. These are usually of the intense variety such as petrol, acetone, or strong perfume. During an attack smells may aggravate the headache and rarely hyperosmia is reported, persisting beyond the headache phase. Although there are few reported studies of olfactory disorder in migraine the connection is believable as it is analogous to the well-established phenomena of photophobia and phonophobia.

Multiple Sclerosis

Pathologically, there is evidence of demyelination in the olfactory tracts and in the periventricular region of the temporal lobes so that hyposmia in this disorder would not be surprising. On the basis of UPSIT-40 and OEP about 15–20% of MS patients have some impairment of smell sense. Sometimes patients report abrupt deterioration of smell sense during a relapse, with recovery either spontaneously or following steroid treatment. Recently it has been shown that hyposmia correlates with the number of cortical plaques measured by MRI.

Tumors and Inflammatory Disease

Within the cranium the olfactory groove menin-gioma is the most common benign tumor and causes anosmia by pressure on the olfactory tract, which lies in the olfactory groove (Figure 3-5). In the early phase, anosmia (if present) is rarely de-tected, as the patient does not notice unilateral anosmia and the clinician, if he tests for it at all, will be even less likely to examine each nostril individu-ally. The main malignant tumor is the temporal lobe glioma producing uncinate fits described in the previous section (see Figure 3-4). Because the tumor is unilateral and many of the temporal lobe functions are duplicated contralaterally it may reach a large size before clinical presentation, par-ticularly if it involves the nondominant side. There is usually no anosmia because the olfactory tracts project to both temporal lobes and olfactory areas in the opposite temporal lobe will compensate.

Miscellaneous Causes

Superficial siderosis, a chronic basal meningitic process, is caused by deposition of hemosiderin on the meninges and can involve the olfactory tract. Such patients are usually deaf and ataxic. In Ref-sum's disease the typical features are polyneuropa-thy, ichthyosis, deafness, and retinitis pigmentosa.

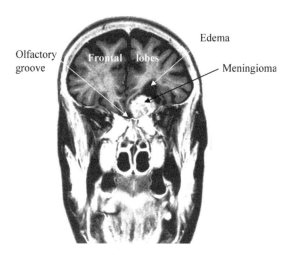

Figure 3-5. Coronal MRI brain scan to show olfactory grove meningioma on left. The dark region above the tumor is edema. This was a 75-year-old woman who, unknown to her, was anosmic just on the left side.

It is less well recognized that most patients with Refsum's syndrome are anosmic. Impaired smell appreciation is occasionally seen in lymphoma and paraneoplastic disorder.

In summary, perceptual olfactory disease may be related to distortion of odor (dysosmia) or hypersensitivity to smells (hyperosmia). Delusions and hallucinations may both occur in the context of epilepsy and psychiatric disease. Many drugs are alleged to cause hyposmia but several claimed associations are anecdotal. The best evidence for anosmia from chemical exposure relates to those compounds directly entering the nasal cavity such as industrial organic chemicals. The most frequent smell loss is the conductive variety followed by viral infection and head injury. Both major and minor head injury can cause smell impairment and the prognosis for recovery is poor overall. Degenerative neurological disease causes olfactory disturbance, notably Alzheimer's and Parkinson's diseases. Less frequently, hyposmia occurs in epilepsy, multiple sclerosis, tumors, and inflammatory nasal disease. Migraine is associated with hyperosmia on rare occasion.

SUGGESTED READING

Amoore JE. Effects of chemical exposure on olfaction in humans. In CS Barrow (ed), Toxicology of the Nasal Passages. Boston: McGraw Hill; 1986:155–190.

Bacon AW, Bondi MW, Salmon DP, Murphy C. Very early changes in olfactory functioning due to Alzheimer's disease and the role of apolipoprotein E in olfaction. Ann N Y Acad Sci 1998;855:723–731.

Barz S, Hummel T, Pauli E, Majer M, Lang CJ, Kobal G. Chemosensory event-related potentials in response to trigeminal and olfactory stimulation in idiopathic Parkinson's disease. Neurology 1997;49:1424–1431.

Berendse HW, Booij J, Francot CM, et al. Subclinical dopaminergic dysfunction in asymptomatic Parkinson's disease patients' relatives with a decreased sense of smell. Ann Neurol 2001;50:34–41.

Doty RL, Deems DA, Frye RE, Pelberg R, Shapiro A. Olfactory sensitivity, nasal resistance, and autonomic function in patients with multiple chemical sensitivities. Arch Otolaryngol Head Neck Surg 1988;114:1422–1427.

Doty RL, Yousem DM, Pham LT, Kreshak AA, Geckle R, Lee WW. Olfactory dysfunction in patients with head trauma. Arch Neurol 1997;54:1131–1140.

Doty RL, Deems DA, Stellar S. Olfactory dysfunction in parkinsonism: a general deficit unrelated to neurologic signs, disease stage, or disease duration. Neurology 1988;38:1237–1244.

Graves AB, Bowen JD, Rajaram L, et al. Impaired olfaction as a marker for cognitive decline: interaction with apolipoprotein E epsilon4 status. Neurology 1999;22(3):1480–1487.

Hawkes CH. Is Parkinson's disease a primary olfactory disorder? QJM 1999;92:473–480.

Henkin RI. Drug-induced taste and smell disorders: incidence, mechanisms, and management related primarily to treatment of sensory receptor dysfunction. Drug Safety 1994;11:318–377.

Montgomery EB Jr., Baker KB, Lyons K, Koller WC. Abnormal performance on the PD test battery by asymptomatic first-degree relatives. Neurology 1999;52:757–762.

Pryse-Phillips W. Disturbance in the sense of smell in psychiatric patients. Proc Roy Soc Med 1975;68: 472–474.

Seiden AM, Duncan HJ. The diagnosis of a conductive olfactory loss. Laryngoscope 2001;111:9–14.

Wenning GK, Shephard B, Hawkes C, Petruckevitch A, Lees A, Quinn N. Olfactory function in typical parkinsonian syndromes. Acta Neurol Scand 1995; 91:247–250.

Investigation, Treatment, and General Management of Olfactory Disease

INVESTIGATION OF SMELL LOSS

The varieties of tests for smell loss have been described already. Of these, the 12-odor international University of Pennsylvania Smell Identification Test (UPSIT) is probably best for routine clinical purposes. Smell identification perception and threshold tests cannot distinguish conductive from perceptive (sensorineural) anosmia. Conductive anosmia has to be excluded first and this is investigated best by anterior rhinoscopy and nasal endoscopy. These two procedures will miss only about 10% of pathologies. The presence of local nasal disease may be evaluated further by rhinomanometry, ciliary motility, and skin tests, if required. If there is any doubt about the diagnosis a high-resolution computed tomography (CT) scan of the nose and paranasal sinuses should be performed. Ear, nose, and throat (ENT) surgeons prefer CT scanning but magnetic resonance imaging (MRI) is often requested by neurologists in the investigation of anosmia as it delineates the olfactory path both peripherally and centrally—it gives good images of the nose and sinuses as well as the brain itself. It displays well the mucosal lining of the nose and sinuses as well as acceptable definition of bone. MRI sometimes overemphasizes the degree of sinus disease.

Olfactory evoked potential recording provides objective evidence of olfactory function and is an ideal method of measuring sensorineural anosmia. It is of particular value in detecting malingering. Unfortunately, it is a complex procedure and available only in few specialized centers.

If peripheral causes are excluded then MRI is the procedure of choice. It excels in demonstrating vascular and traumatic lesions of the brain and can be adapted to quantitative measurement of the olfactory bulbs and hippocampus. In schizophrenia and diseases with severe perceptive anosmia such as parkinsonism there are no characteristic changes; likewise in Alzheimer's disease there is typically temporoparietal atrophy but no specific lesion in cortical olfactory areas.

If the patient is suspected to be describing an olfactory aura, then epilepsy needs to be considered and electroencephalography and MRI brain scan would be the initial key investigations.

A blood screen should be performed, testing in particular the blood count (for anemia, drug effects); sedimentation rate (vasculitic disease, malignancy); B12 and folate level (nutritional state); glucose (diabetes and pituitary disease); calcium and phosphate (parathyroid function, Paget's disease); thyroid function (myxedema); electrolytes (renal disease, Addison's or Cushing's disease); liver function tests (cirrhosis); autoimmune tests such as antineutrophil cytoplasmic autoantibodies (ANCA) for Wegener's granulomatosis, and anti-Ro and anti-La for Sjögren's disease; and IgE (hay fever). Further investigation depends on complexity and whether there is a question of malingering, as may be the case in compensation claims.

TREATMENT

Therapy directed to the underlying cause is the obvious treatment for local nasal inflammatory disease and tumor whether growing in the sinuses or intra-cranially. Any process that is obstructing the flow of air to the olfactory mucosa should be corrected—either surgically or with steroids or anti-inflammatory spray. Predictably, steroids are used for granulomata affecting the nose such as Wegener's or sarcoidosis. Wegener's granulomatosis usually needs more vigorous immunosuppression than steroids alone can provide (e.g., cyclophosphamide or methotrexate). Recent reports suggest that sulphonamides (e.g., co-trimoxazole) may be just as effective. If hyposmia is associated with nasal polyps steroids may be of considerable value because of their anti-inflammatory and anti-edema effect. They are more beneficial when given systemically than topically. Recent unconfirmed reports suggest that vitamin A might aid recovery in chronic nasal sinus disease. Surgery for polyps is indicated only for very large medically refractory polyps or where there is diagnostic uncertainty.

Steroids have also been tried for the patient hyposmic from head injury. There are no large randomized trials to validate their use. It is conventional to give prednisolone initially in high dose for the first few weeks and then tapering the dose for the following 3 weeks. The rationale is that scarring around the cribriform plate area may impede the growth of centripetal olfactory neurones and connection with the bulb might be reestablished if the scarred tissue can be softened. More likely, any beneficial effect results from reduction in local nasal edema and long-term benefit is dubious. Some use zinc but once more this is not supported by evidence-based medicine and most consider it to be valueless.

Hyperosmia

Treatment of hyperosmia is not easy. Anecdotally, the only compounds that seem to be of benefit are the anti-epileptic preparations. This is a matter of personal choice but many use carbamazepine or sodium valproate. With both compounds it is important to start at low dose and then build up to the maximum tolerable. On basic principles, an anti-depressant might help whether used alone or in conjunction with an anticonvulsant.

MEDICOLEGAL ASPECTS

Head injury is a common cause of anosmia. It can occur on rare occasion with mild trauma in the absence of skull fracture and will be seen occasionally in whiplash injury. Experts working for insurance companies who deal with head-injured patients regularly fail to ask about smell impairment and if any tests are done they are usually inadequate. It is insufficient, even negligent, just to ask patients about their smell perception; it must be tested. In outpatient practice the 12-odor UPSIT or sniffin' sticks are suitable for screening. If abnormality is found, then further evaluation or repeated screening would be appropriate at, say, yearly intervals although the prognosis for recovery is poor overall. If the injury involves the face there may be conductive anosmia from fracture of nasal bones, displacement of the septum, or nasal congestion from blood and debris. This type may resolve after surgical correction and resolution of edema, so further testing is essential.

During recovery there may be distortion of smell perception—everyday odors may taste bland or unpleasant (cacosmia). About one-third of those in this group improve slowly but in the rest it is permanent. Treatment is unsatisfactory but drugs mentioned earlier for hyperosmia (anti-epileptics or antidepressants) should be tried. Hyperosmia itself after head injury is extremely rare.

According to guidance given by Sumner, courts will wish to satisfy themselves on several counts:

- That trauma or industrial exposure can produce anosmia itself—a now incontrovertible fact.
- That there was no evidence of anosmia before the episode.

- That local causes of anosmia have been excluded.
- That there is no sign of amplification of symptoms or frank malingering.
- That the prognosis for recovery is based on reasoned assessment.

It is sometimes difficult to know when to finalize a claim for anosmia as there is prospect for recovery after a long period. In broad terms, an interval of 5 years from date of injury would be reasonable. If smell sense has not recovered by then it is likely to be permanent. The exception as mentioned earlier is parosmia, which can recover in about one-third of cases over 8 years. Few people are happy to wait that long and one may have to compromise by serial assessment to determine the point at which no further improvement has taken place.

Detection of the malingerer is particularly problematic in cases of personal injury where the potential compensation is large; the prevalence of malingering was 14% in one series. The use of strong ammonia for alleged anosmics is a favorite but crude procedure. A true anosmic will report the trigeminal burning effect of ammonia but the malingerer may deny even that. The clever malingerer may be smart enough to report the irritant effect, making the test not particularly reliable. One approach described by Kurtz and colleagues involves the so-called olfactory confusion matrix. This requires the identification of 10 test odors in 100 trials of which two (vinegar and ammonia) are strongly trigeminal. It is based on the assumption that malingerers believe that they should demonstrate loss of smell to all compounds irrespective of their strengths and trigeminal effects. They found that volunteers who tried to simulate malingering rarely reported a trigeminal (irritant) attribute in 10 trials of vinegar whereas the true anosmic usually did. Unfortunately, the differences were not absolute or statistically significant and could not detect reliably the person who was amplifying his or her symptoms or the malingerer who was knowledgeable about trigeminal effects. Suspicions may be aroused likewise if the subject scores unusually low on UPSIT. Malingerers will return a score of 0–5, for example, on the 40-odor booklets or by extrapolation 0–1 on the 12-odor book, probably because they deliberately deselect the correct answer. Microsmic individuals scratch the UPSIT test strip more vigorously than anosmic or normal people and this feature might be of help to spot the malingerer. Another test involves the "method of magnitude estimation," which basically compares the relationship between concentration and perceived intensity. The log of these variables should produce a straight line. Someone with pollutant exposure has a flat slope (i.e., large increases of concentration are required to produce small increments in perceived intensity). A non-linear relationship would arouse suspicion. To complicate matters further, it has been suggested that anosmic patients have decreased sensitivity to trigeminal stimulation. Objective tests of olfaction such as the olfactory evoked response are ideally situated to this situation. Brain imaging MRI, CT, or single photon emission computerized tomography (SPECT) may show post-traumatic change in a relevant area such as the insular or orbitofrontal cortex or temporal lobe, and in males there may be atrophy of the olfactory bulb. Specialist referral is mandatory for suspected malingerers.

The medicolegal, and indeed everyday clinical, importance of anosmia or hyposmia relates to a person's occupation. A wine taster or chef will be unemployable if there is even the smallest reduction in olfactory identification or threshold and their potential for legitimate financial compensation is high. This contrasts with the unskilled laborer, who would be entitled to far less. The laborer's work should be allowed to continue in most instances unless a good sense of smell was essential and the person had to work alone. A retired person likewise would command less financial reward, but the dangers in everyday life must not be underestimated nor the lack of enjoyment of food or drink and the overall reduction in the quality of life.

On the industrial front there are a large number of olfactory toxins that may cause damage, as listed in Table 3-3. Unquestionably, there is an association between many of those listed but several reports are anecdotal or based on small numbers in financially motivated individuals. Some odor complaints about pollutants are simply a result of the sensory properties of the pollutants themselves rather than direct pathological change in the olfactory receptor or neural pathway. Persons exposed to pollutants may be receiving or have taken medication that in itself can affect smell sense or they may suffer coexisting disease known to alter olfaction. Note should be made of the compound alleged to have caused the olfactory defect and whether several substances were involved simultaneously. For most compounds there is a published threshold limit volume (TLV) that gives an idea of maximum safe exposure levels and from this the magnitude of exposure can be estimated. This is of most relevance in cases of acute exposure but for chronic exposure there may be individual susceptibility. The duration of exposure, latency of onset to first symptoms, their progression, and whether there is dysosmia need to be recorded as well as the quality of ventilation and filtration and whether one or more workers had comparable symptoms at the same time.

GENERAL ADVICE AND
VOCATIONAL ISSUES

Anosmic patients and even those experiencing natural decline of smell function through aging should be given guidance on simple precautions. A significant number of elderly die from gas poisoning each year. Consumption of infected food probably causes minor ailments in the elderly and on occasion food poisoning. Nutritional problems and weight loss in the aged may relate to anosmia as food loses its appeal. Indeed it is suspected that the frequent finding of weight loss in patients with advanced Parkinson's disease relates to hyposmia, which as mentioned earlier affects 80% of patients. A smoke detector is essential for the kitchen and in every room where there is a fireplace. It is preferable to have a detector in all bedrooms, particularly in those belonging to smokers. An electric stove is preferable to a gas stove. If gas is installed patients should purchase a detector for this as well. Propane, butane, and gasoline are heavier than air and because of this detectors for them should be placed near the ground. Natural gas and smoke are lighter than air, so the detectors for these need to be placed near the ceiling or top of the stairwell. Anosmic persons may have difficulty detecting spoiled food that can be hazardous to eat. They should be encouraged to discard leftover food and ideally ask someone with normal smell sense to check all food before consumption. Finally, advice should be given on how to enhance the appeal of food with artificial flavorings, which increase the smell and taste of food. In so doing appetite is improved and the common tendency to weight loss or even malnutrition is avoided.

In summary, treatment of olfactory disorder is directed to the underlying disease. Zinc supplements are extensively tried but their value is dubious. Steroids are beneficial for local nasal conditions particularly where there is conductive anosmia from polyps or hay fever. When compensation is being sought the patient is best directed to a unit specializing in assessment of medicolegal problems. It is important to give patients general advice about their occupations, safety in the home, and how to make food more palatable and safe to eat.

SUGGESTED READING

Doty RL, Genow A, Hummel T. Scratch density differentiates microsmic from normosmic and anosmic subjects on the University of Pennsylvania Smell Identification Test. Percept Mot Skills 1998;86: 211–216.
Kurtz DB, White TL, Hornung DE, Belknap E. What a tangled web we weave: discriminating between

malingering and anosmia. Chem Senses 1999;24: 697–700.

Stegeman CA, Cohen Tervaert JW, de Jong PE, Kallenberg CG. Trimethoprim-sulfamethoxazole (co-trimoxazole) for the prevention of relapses of Wegener's granulomatosis. Dutch Co-Trimoxazole Wegener Study Group. N Engl J Med 1996;335: 16–20.

Sumner D. Disturbances of the senses of smell and taste after head injuries. In PJ Vinken, GW Bruyn (eds), Handbook of Neurology. Vol 24. Injuries of the Brain and Skull Part II. Amsterdam: Elsevier, 1976: 1–25.

Taste

Anatomy and Physiology of Taste Sense

INTRODUCTION

Taste is the least studied human sensory modality and much of the scientific literature relates to animal work. Very few clinical neurologists have a research interest in taste so that detailed clinical data are frequently lacking. On the basis of the National Health Interview Survey of about 80,000 adults it was estimated that when adjusted for age, there would be 1.1 million Americans (0.6%) with a taste problem. This contrasts with 2.7 million estimated to have a chronic olfactory problem. Age was a major factor, with those over 65 years accounting for 40% of those with disability. In the University of

Pennsylvania Smell & Taste Center, taste complaints were dwarfed by olfactory complaints, only 4% of patients with chemosensory complaints presenting with such a problem, but this may relate in part to patients' expectation of useful treatment. Despite such compelling prevalence data, the assessment of taste is frequently neglected by clinicians.

A definition of terms is required and is summarized in Table 5-1: *ageusia* is loss of taste; *hypogeusia* is diminution in taste; *dysgeusia* is distortion of taste; *hypergeusia* is increased taste perception. The olfactory equivalents of cacosmia (cacogeusia), phantosmia (phantogeusia), parosmia (parageusia), osmophobia (gustatophobia), and torquosmia (torquegeusia) are rarely used descriptors. In *heterogeusia* everything tastes the same and this appears a common complaint in dyspeptic patients. Once again *homogeusia* would be a preferable term. *Presbygeusia* is the natural age-related decline of taste appreciation. Some divide taste impairment into three categories: type 1 is absence of stimulus recognition with varying degrees of taste detection; type 2 is decreased ability to detect or recognize stimuli; and type 3 is decreased ability to judge stimulus intensity with normal detection and recognition thresholds.

Table 5-1. Definition of various terms to describe taste abnormalities

Term	Definition
Ageusia	Absence of taste sense
Hypogeusia or microgeusia	Reduction of taste sense
Dysgeusia	Distortion of taste sense
Parageusia	Distortion due to a specific stimulus
Phantogeusia	Distortion when there is no external stimulus
Cacogeusia	Unpleasant type of distortion
Torquegeusia	Burning type of distortion
Hypergeusia	Increased sensitivity to common taste
Gustatophobia	Dislike of certain tastes
Heterogeusia	All food and drink taste the same
Presbygeusia	Decline of taste sense with age
Type 1 hypogeusia	Inability to recognize stimulus with varying degrees of detection
Type 2 hypogeusia	Decreased detection or recognition
Type 3 hypogeusia	Reduced intensity ability with normal detection and recognition

ANATOMY AND PHYSIOLOGY

Receptors for taste are distributed throughout the tongue and to lesser degree over the rest of the oral cavity, pharynx, and esophagus. A taste bud consists of a clump of receptor cells at microscopic level that form visible swellings or papillae of four varieties named after their shape: circumvallate, meaning a battlement surrounded by a moat; foliate, or leaf-shaped; filiform, or thread-shaped; and fungiform, mushroom-shaped (Figure 5-1). Each bud has a central pore at the apex to allow entry of liquid. The circumvallate and large fungiform papillae are found in the root of the tongue whereas the foliate papillae occupy the posterolateral margins. The dorsal surface of the tongue is mainly occupied by filiform papillae with interspersed smaller fungiform papillae. There are an estimated 4600 taste buds in the human tongue and their cells regenerate roughly every 10 days, but this process does not include their axons.

Excluding autonomic supply, the nose has a nerve supply from two cranial nerves (I and V) but the tongue receives input from four—V, VII, IX, and X—of which three are directly concerned with taste, so there is considerable spare capacity. Common sensation such as touch, pain, and temperature is provided over the anterior two-thirds by the trigem-

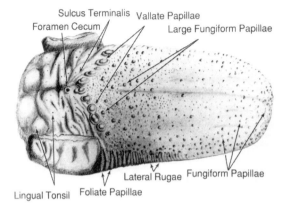

Figure 5-1. Surface anatomy of the tongue. (Reprinted with permission from Miller IJ. Anatomy of the peripheral taste system. In RL Doty (ed), Handbook of Olfaction and Gustation. New York: Marcel Dekker Inc., 1995; Chapter 23.)

inal nerve through its lingual branch. The posterior one-third and adjacent soft palate are fed by the glossopharyngeal nerve (Color Plate 5A). Taste perception for the anterior two-thirds is through the chorda tympani, which joins the facial nerve in the middle ear. The chorda tympani also contains secretomotor fibers destined for the submandibular and sublingual salivary glands so that a lesion of this nerve will impair taste twice by damaging visceral afferent fibers and causing the mouth to become dry. The posterior third of the tongue for taste and common sensation is also supplied by the glossopharyngeal nerve, the afferent fibers of which ascend to the inferior ganglion of IX and then into the medulla. The relatively fewer taste buds in the epiglottis, larynx, and upper third of the esophagus are supplied by branches of the vagus (Color Plate 5A). Salivation, which is indirectly related to the ability to taste, is controlled by the superior and inferior salivatory nuclei (located in the rostral part of the dorsal vagal nucleus in the medulla) through fibers that join the chorda tympani and glossopharyngeal nerves. The sensitivity of the human taste receptor is reasonable in that 0.05 mg/dL (1 part in 2000) of quinine sulphate will produce a bitter taste but is nowhere approaching that of the olfactory system.

The three taste nerves terminate in the nucleus of the solitary tract (NST), a linear structure in the medulla that is sandwiched between the spinal nucleus of V laterally and the dorsal nucleus of X medially (Color Plate 5B). Fibers from the chorda tympani terminate in its rostral section; IX terminates in the mid-portion and X in the caudal part so that taste-wise the tongue is arranged in a rostro-caudal fashion in the NST with the tip of the tongue the most superior part. Nonprimates have an indirect thalamic taste projection that relays in the pons (parabrachial nuclei) but in the human there is a monosynaptic uncrossed projection direct to the thalamus. The thalamic gustatory nucleus is the parvicellular portion of ventroposteromedial nucleus (VPMpc), essentially a medial extension of VPM that receives the main trigeminal input (Color Plate 5B). From VPMpc there is projection to the frontal operculum and insular cortex that is probably the primary cortical taste center and logically it is situated close to the tongue in the primary motor cortex. Projections go from these areas to a secondary taste area in the orbitofrontal cortex and from there to the amygdala and lateral hypothalamus (i.e., joining the limbic system). Olfactory signals also reach the orbitofrontal cortex (mainly on the right side) so this zone integrates taste, vision, olfaction, and probably touch (Figure 5-2). Functional MRI (fMRI) studies confirm this projection and show activation in the frontal operculum, insula, and orbitofrontal cortices for both olfactory and taste stimulation. Positron emission tomography (PET) studies show increased blood flow in the amygdala and left orbitofrontal cortex during exposure to offensive odorants and tastants.

A difficulty with human functional imaging is that inadvertently most taste stimulants used activate the common sensory part of the lingual nerve and therefore the derived cortical representation

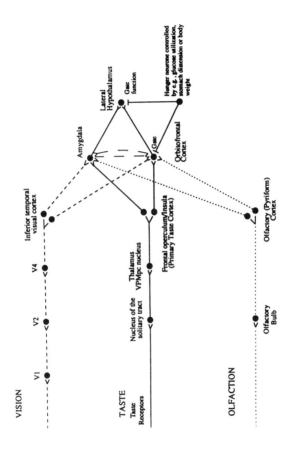

Figure 5-2. Central taste pathways showing how they converge centrally with olfactory and visual pathways. VPMpc = ventroposteromedial thalamic nucleus, parvicellular region. V1, V2, and V4 are visual cortical areas. (Reprinted with permission from Rolls ET. Central taste anatomy and neurophysiology. In RL Doty (ed), Handbook of Olfaction and Gustation. New York: Marcel Dekker Inc., 1995; Chapter 24.)

may be coupled with that for common sensation of the tongue as well as taste. It is probable that taste signals are represented bilaterally in the cerebral cortex, although the main projection from medulla and thalamus is ipsilateral and most likely the left cortex is dominant for taste recognition in right-handed people. The orbitofrontal cortex also receives information about the sight of objects and faces from the amygdala and cortical visual areas. Neurons therein learn the visual stimuli associated with reinforcing (pleasant) tastes but the reverse pattern can be acquired (i.e., aversion to unpleasant tastes or visual signals). The central convergence of taste, smell, and visual information at the cortical level possibly explains in part why so many purely anosmic patients complain that they have lack of taste and have difficulty distinguishing smell from taste loss.

The classical primary varieties of taste are sweet, sour, salt, and bitter. According to traditional teaching salt and sweet are located at the front, sour on the lateral border, and bitter at the rear of the tongue. Some maintain that sour and bitter perceptions are best appreciated over the palate. Recently, a fifth primary taste has been proposed called *umami*, a Japanese word meaning delicious or savory, which is elicited by the taste of L-glutamate, the main component of monosodium glutamate. If a mixture of monosodium glutamate and ribonucleotides is consumed it is described variously as brothy, soupy, meaty, or savory.

Transduction is the process of changing the energy of the stimulant (here taste) into electro-chemical energy to form an action potential. A diagram of taste transduction mechanism is shown in Figure 5-3. Sour and salt tastes are transduced mainly by ion channels located at the apex of the taste receptor cell. Amiloride (the diuretic) is a sodium channel blocker and many reports show that amiloride diminishes the intensity of sodium chloride taste when applied to the tip of the tongue, possibly by decreasing its sourness. The antiseptic chlorhexidine, known to block sodium channels, reduces the saltiness of various salts but less so the bitterness of several compounds. In ciguatera poisoning a metallic taste is sometimes experienced that may relate to the ability of the ciguatera toxin to block sodium channels in the tongue. Sour taste is mediated by hydrogen ions and transduced by receptor cells located mainly in the posterior and lateral border of the tongue (fungiform, foliate, and circumvallate papillae).

Sweet and bitter taste are mainly transduced by receptors coupled to G proteins (in similar fashion to olfactory transduction) that exert their effects through second messengers acting on specific intracellular targets such as kinases or basolateral

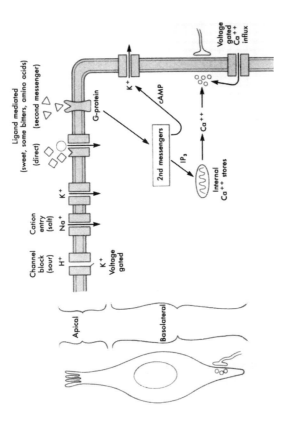

Figure 5-3. Transduction pathway for taste receptors. Some sour and bitter substances are transduced by the closing of apical voltage-sensitive potassium channels. Transduction of salts such as sodium chloride involves movement of ions like sodium and potassium through amiloride-sensitive cation channels in the apical membrane. Sweet and some bitter compounds are thought to activate intracellular second messenger pathways such as cyclic adenosine monophosphate (cAMP) and inositol triphosphate (IP$_3$), which leads to activation of membrane channels in the basolateral membrane of the taste cell. (Reprinted with permission from Sweazey RD. Olfaction and taste. In DE Haines (ed), Fundamental Neuroscience. Philadelphia: Churchill Livingstone, 1997; Chapter 22.)

channels. A recently discovered G protein known as alpha-gustducin (structurally related to rod and cone transducin in the retina) is probably concerned with bitter and sweet perception. Sweet taste can be blocked by gymnema tea or lactisole but the mechanism of action is unclear. Interestingly, gymnema tea has been used as an Indian folk remedy for diabetes as it slows the absorption of sugar in the gut, reduces the sweet taste of food, and acts as an appetite suppressant. Sodium salts and a mixture of lactoglobulin with phosphatidic acid will block the bitterness of caffeine or quinine. Blockers for acid sourness and umami tastes are not known as yet. Umami taste is thought to be transduced by both receptors and apical ion channels (see Figure 5-3). Synaptic neurotransmitters or neuromodulators released at synapses in taste buds have not yet been identified with certainty. The best evidence is for serotonin but adrenergic, cholinergic, and peptidergic transmitters may also be involved.

Studies in gene knockout mice show that the development of taste buds and somatic tongue innervation is heavily dependent on two growth factors: brain-derived neurotrophic factor (BDNF) and neurotrophin 3 (NT3). If BDNF is not expressed there is a reduction in taste bud number and impaired taste perception. If NT3 is missing there is severe loss of somatosensory innervation to the mouth and tongue. It is probable that a taste bud will not develop until it has a nerve supply, so that these two growth factors are interdependent. Deficiency of BDNF may have relevance to familial dysautonomia (see following section) where there is loss of taste and marked reduction of taste bud number. A third growth factor, essential at least in rodents, mischievously termed "sonic hedgehog," is probably important for the development of taste buds and their pattern. So far no gustatory disease due to deficiency of sonic hedgehog is described in humans but it probably will soon.

FUNCTION OF SALIVA

Saliva has a dominant role in taste appreciation. Without moisture, which allows chewed-up food to be conveyed to the taste buds for analysis, there is no taste. Drying of the mouth, seen in Sjögren's syndrome, is associated with ageusia, likewise as in cystic fibrosis where saliva is more viscous. Saliva is able to digest starch through salivary amylase that in turn produces a mildly sweet taste. Phenylthio-carbamide (PTC) has a bitter taste (see Taste Threshold and Taste Blindness section later in this chapter) that is not universally perceived, and the ability to detect it has been claimed to depend on the chemical constitution of an individual's saliva. Sucrose octa-acetate (SOA) has a bitter taste and has been extensively studied in the mouse. Close linkage of mouse genes for SOA bitter taste perception and salivary proline-rich proteins (PRP) has been found. This is of interest as such genes are highly conserved between mouse and human and because there is a high level of PRP in human saliva, all of which would suggest that there might be a gene for bitterness shared by mice and man. PRPs have the ability to bind with tannins (bitter) so that food may become more palatable as a result of this reaction, although not necessarily safer. The perception of saltiness probably depends on ambient concentrations of sodium and potassium in saliva to which taste cells adapt. This process possibly determines the threshold to various salts. Sourness relates to the pH of saliva and its buffering capacity.

Saliva contains small quantities of a zinc-metalloprotein that was initially called gustin but has subsequently been found to be identical to carbonic anhydrase VI. Zinc deficiency that may impair taste could produce its effects via this compound. If the rate of saliva production is diminished, the health of the mouth is reduced and patients complain of pain, burning, and metallic taste. Many drugs are excreted into saliva and produce a metallic or other unpleasant taste: these include tetracyclines, captopril, lithium carbonate, and penicillamine (see Table 7-1).

TASTE THRESHOLD AND TASTE BLINDNESS

The threshold for stimulation of sour by hydrochloric acid is on average 0.0009M; for salt by sodium chloride 0.01M; for sweet by sucrose 0.01M; and for bitter by quinine 0.000008M. Thus the threshold for bitter is much lower and this has probably developed for protective purposes because most poisonous substances have a bitter taste. Not all bitter or sour substances have the same intensity, and the relative degree of bitterness/sourness has been measured. The threshold to a given taste varies according to its quality (bitter, sour, etc.) as well as the nature of the chemical itself (Figure 5-4).

The term *taste blindness* or *specific ageusia* refers to inherited lack of taste detection for certain chemicals in the presence of preserved taste for other compounds and is comparable to specific anosmia and color blindness. In contrast to smell blindness, there are few examples of specific ageusia so far described in humans. Despite this, inherited ageusia is of major interest because of the prospect that

Sour Substances	Index	Bitter Substances	Index	Sweet Substances	Index	Salty Substances	Index
Hydrochloric acid	1	Quinine	1	Sucrose	1	NaCl	1
Formic acid	1.1	Brucine	11	1-propoxy-2-amino-4-nitrobenzene	5000	NaF	2
Chloracetic acid	0.9	Strychnine	3.1	Saccharin	675	CaCl₂	1
Acetyllactic acid	0.85	Nicotine	1.3	Chloroform	40	NaBr	0.4
Lactic acid	0.85	Phenylthiourea	0.9	Fructose	1.7	NaI	0.35
Tartaric acid	0.7	Caffeine	0.4	Alanine	1.3	LiCl	0.4
Malic acid	0.6	Veratrine	0.2	Glucose	0.8	NH₄Cl	2.5
Potassium H tartrate	0.58	Pilocarpine	0.16	Maltose	0.45	KCl	0.6
Acetic acid	0.55	Atropine	0.13	Galactose	0.32		
Citric acid	0.46	Cocaine	0.02	Lactose	0.3		
Carbonic acid	0.06	Morphine	0.02				

Figure 5-4. Relative taste indices (the reciprocal of thresholds) of various substances. The intensities of the four primary sensations of taste are referred respectively to the intensities of taste of hydrochloric acid, quinine, sucrose, and sodium chloride, each of which is considered to have a taste index of 1. (Reprinted with permission from Guyton AC, Hall JE. Textbook of Medical Physiology (9th ed). Philadelphia: WB Saunders, 1996:676.)

genetic studies might lead to the identification of specific taste receptors and their associated genes. The most frequently studied agent has been PTC, which tastes bitter to some and bland to others. This specific ageusia is inherited as an autosomal recessive trait and is most common in whites (30%), followed by Orientals (10%), then Afro-Caribbeans (3%). PTC non-tasters are insensitive to several other bitter compounds such as propylthiouracil (PROP) the antithyroid agent. Such people are inadvertently liable to consume isothiocyanates and goitrin, which are bitter-tasting compounds found in vegetables such as cabbage, broccoli, and brussels sprouts. More recently, supertasters to PROP have been identified in 25% of healthy Americans who have a higher than average number of fungiform papillae. Interestingly, PTC and PROP tasters have a lower incidence of thyroid deficiency, suggesting that they have a biological advantage; they are more sensitive to the bitterness or burning of caffeine, potassium chloride, capsaicin (chili pepper), and saccharin but not to quinine. They are also more sensitive than non-tasters to the sweet taste of saccharin and sucrose. However, both tasters and non-tasters detect the bitter taste of quinine at normal threshold levels, suggesting that the perception of bitterness is governed by several receptors, each with their respective genes.

Most recently it has been suggested that some people are non-tasters to either glucose or fructose. In one study of 92 subjects there were 12 non-tasters to glucose and 4 to fructose. Repeated exposure of non-tasters to glucose improved their response in parallel with the improved sensitivity found in those initially smell blind to androsterone (see Smell section). Probably many more instances of taste blindness remain to be discovered in humans, and this will probably follow studies of knockout gene models in rodents.

There are two rival theories for coding of taste quality: the "across fiber" theory and the "labelled line" hypothesis. In the across fiber theory it is proposed that quality is coded by the pattern of activity across neurons. The labelled line hypothesis suggests that taste neuron types are specific coding channels for taste quality. Individual taste receptor cells probably do not code for just one class of tastants in humans, although they do in some invertebrates and fish. More likely they code for several stimulant classes (across fiber or broad tuning) although it is suspected that they show preference for one class over another. There is probably some crude taste appreciation from bare lingual nerve endings located on the tongue surface and because of central convergence there are thalamic neurons that respond to both taste and touch signals. There is also considerable modification of afferent taste signals both peripherally and centrally.

CONDITIONED TASTE AVERSION

The decision whether to eat a food or not depends on the ability to discriminate between various tastants. Animals and humans can be taught to avoid certain flavors by pairing the taste with gastrointestinal malaise. Following such learning the degree to which aversion applies to other stimuli can indicate the taste similarity of various tastants. For example, an animal taught to avoid sucrose, without conditioning, will also avoid fructose, glucose, and saccharin. Some reactions are thought to be innate, not requiring conditioning. For example, premature babies show pleasure with sweet tastes and dislike for bitter tastes in the absence of prior experience. It is presumed that this response is hard wired into the nervous system for protection in that many harmful substances are bitter tasting.

Beyond the initial predisposition, preferences can be strengthened or weakened by repeated exposure. On first sampling, chili is found unpleasant and burning in quality. Through repeated exposure some people come to like it even though it still burns! The palatability of a compound may vary according to satiety. For example, when a sweet substance is eaten it is initially reported as pleasant but on repeated exposure (as long as the sweet substance is swallowed) the taste becomes unpleasant. Conditioning may play a role in the weight loss associated with anorexia nervosa, cancer, or depression. One theory suggests that in anorexia nervosa increased production of estrogen at puberty causes food aversion. Indeed there is evidence in animals that estrogens suppress appetite. Taste preference and aversion probably relate to plastic changes in taste-responsive cells in the orbitofrontal cortex and their connections with the amygdala and visual cortex (see Figure 5-2).

In summary, taste is detected by receptor cells located within various papillae on the surface of the tongue. The orthodox primary tastes of sweet, sour, bitter, and salt have been supplemented by a fifth known as umami. Transduction is achieved by ion channels or G-receptor proteins. Three nerves transmit taste sensation (chorda tympani, glossopharyngeal, and vagus) to the nucleus of the solitary tract and on to the VPMpc in the thalamus, insula, and orbitofrontal cortex. Coding of taste quality in humans depends on interaction of neurons concerned with specific tastants and the pattern they evoke rather than signalling from specialized taste receptors. Saliva is essential for taste both in quantity and quality. Some people are born with inability to detect two bitter compounds—PTC and PROP—and two sweet compounds—glucose and fructose. This, and conditioning both innate and learned, may influence personal likes and dislikes in food.

SUGGESTED READING

Bartoshuk LM, Duffy VB, Miller IJ. PTC/PROP tasting: anatomy, psychophysics, and sex effects. Physiol Behav 1994;56:1165–1171.

Bernstein IL. Taste aversion learning: a contemporary perspective. Nutrition 1999;15:229–234.

Hoffman HJ, Ishii EK, MacTurk RH. Age-related changes in the prevalence of smell/taste problems among the United States adult population. Results of the 1994 disability supplement to the National Health Interview Survey (NHIS). Ann N Y Acad Sci 1998; 855:716–722.

Kaplan MD, Baum BJ. The functions of saliva. Dysphagia 1993;8:225–229.

Rolls ET. Central taste anatomy and neurophysiology. In RL Doty (ed), Handbook of Olfaction and Gustation. New York: Marcel Dekker Inc., 1995;549–573.

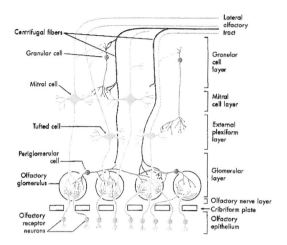

Color Plate 1 Schematic drawing of the olfactory bulb showing the laminar organization, major cell types, and basic circuitry. Receptor neurons are shown in blue, interneurons in red, the efferent neurons of the bulb in green, and centrifugal fibers in black. (Reprinted with permission from Sweazey RD. Olfaction and taste. In DE Haines (ed), Fundamental Neuroscience. Philadelphia: Churchill Livingstone, 1997; Chapter 22.)

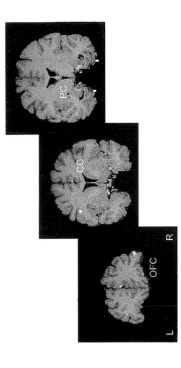

Color Plate 2 Olfactory fMRI at 3.0 T. Areas of activation due to the vanillin odorant for one representative subject overlaid on MPRAGE images. Coronal sections at an uncorrected probability p<0.001. OFC = Orbitofrontal Cortex; CC = Cingulate Cortex; PC = Piriform Cortex. (Reprinted with permission from Kettenmann B, Francis S, Aspen J, et al. Repeated trigeminal stimuli result in a constant or even sensitized SII activity while olfactory-related activity generally shows attenuation. Chem Sens 2001;26(8):1085–1086.)

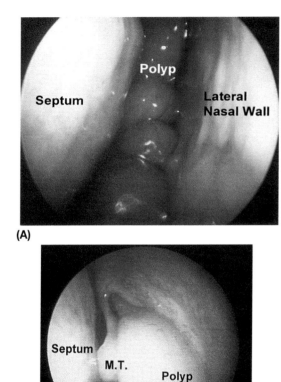

(A)

(B)

Color Plates 3A–C Photographs of various types of polyps as seen through nasal endoscope. M.T. represents middle turbinate. (Courtesy of Mr. H. Kaddour.)

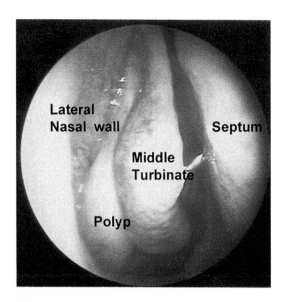

(C)

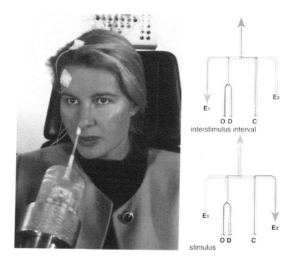

Color Plate 4 Bottom left: recording setup showing a thin piece of Teflon tubing inserted into the nose. Bottom right: technique of creating a bolus of odorant without disturbing the main airflow. The main odorless air C (in blue) is continually blown into the nose in resting conditions (upper diagram). The airstream-containing odor (O, in red) is sucked away by vacuum E1. To achieve an olfactory stimulus, the odorless air C is vented away by vacuum E2 while simultaneously E1 is closed. This allows the odor-containing gas to reach the nose imperceptibly without disturbing the main inflow and therefore avoiding trigeminal stimulation.

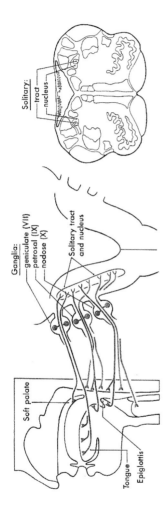

Color Plate 5A   The main three nerves concerned with taste and their connection to the solitary tract nucleus in the medulla. Special visceral afferent fibers (red) terminate in the rostral (gustatory) areas of the solitary nucleus. General visceral afferent fibers (blue) terminate in the caudal portion of the nucleus.

Ganglia:
geniculate (VII)
petrosal (IX)
nodose (X)

Solitary tract and nucleus

Soft palate

Tongue

Epiglottis

Solitary:
tract
nucleus

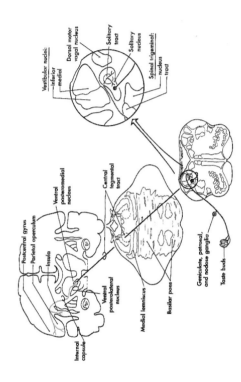

Color Plate 5B The ascending taste pathway from medulla to cortex. (Reprinted with permission from Sweazey RD. Olfaction and taste. In DE Haines (ed), Fundamental Neuroscience. Philadelphia: Churchill Livingstone, 1997; Chapter 22.)

Labels on figure:

Vestibular nuclei:
- inferior
- medial

Dorsal motor vagal nucleus

Solitary tract

Solitary nucleus

Spinal trigeminal:
- nucleus
- tract

Postcentral gyrus

Parietal operculum

Insula

Ventral posteromedial nucleus

Central tegmental tract

Ventral posterolateral nucleus

Internal capsule

Medial lemniscus

Basilar pons

Geniculate, petrosal, and nodose ganglia

Taste buds

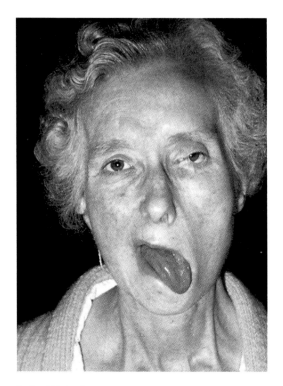

Color Plate 6 Patient with advanced glomus jugulare tumor. This woman presented with left conductive deafness followed by lesions of the 5th to 12th cranial nerves. Note the smooth left brow, the tarsorrhaphy to protect the anesthetic eye. There is wasting of the left sternomastoid (XI) and deviation of the tongue (XII) to left because of a left 12th nerve palsy. (Reprinted with permission from Parsons M. A Colour Atlas of Neurology (2nd ed). London: Wolfe Publishing, 1993.)

Clinical Assessment of Taste

HISTORY AND EXAMINATION

As in smell disorder, patients infrequently volunteer a problem with taste appreciation and when they do it often indicates a disorder of smell sense. Once more the patient has to be asked specifically if there is a problem. Note should be made of the onset, duration, drug or chemical exposure, nutritional status, smoking habit, and type of taste disorder (e.g., distorted or lost).

It is essential to examine the tongue, dentures/teeth, and pharynx for sign of infection. Particular note should be made of the fungiform papillae as their number will be reduced in a variety of autonomic neuropathies. If methylene blue is applied to

147

Table 6-1. Checklist for history taking in patients complaining of taste problem

Is taste problem intermittent or continuous?

Onset: sudden or gradual; bilateral or unilateral?

Is smell also affected?

Does eating mask the taste distortion or does the distortion mask the enjoyment of food?

Can anything be tasted at all?

Any precipitating event such as surgery or trauma?

Are there bad tastes without a stimulus (phantogeusia) or with a stimulus (parageusia) and what is the taste like?

Is there facial numbness, dysphagia, hoarseness, pain on swallowing, aspiration, choking, dry mouth or dry eyes?

Is there pain, burning, numbness, or soreness in tongue? Any vesicles on tongue?

Is there previous history of trauma, surgery, radiation, or tumor? Get details of head injury—fracture, loss and duration of loss of consciousness.

Is there history of Bell's palsy?

Past medical health—especially diabetes, endocrine disease?

Systems review.

Social and occupational history for smoking, work exposure to toxins.

Modified with permission from Cullen MM, Leopold DA. Disorders of smell and taste. Med Clin North Am 1999;83:57–74.

Table 6-2. Checklist for main areas to be assessed in patients with a taste problem

Region	Main Observations and Tests
Ears	Serous otitis media indicating naso-pharyngeal mass or inflammation Status of middle ear and evidence of previous surgery Hearing tests
Nose	Anterior rhinoscopy for nasal mass
Eyes	Dry eyes. Schirmer strip test
Oral cavity	Nasopharyngeal mass Check tongue for: number, size, distribution of papillae Health of mucosae Presence, quantity, and quality of saliva State of teeth, gums, and tonsils
Neck	Palpate for masses, thyroid enlargement, previous neck surgery Palpate salivary glands for tenderness or masses
Nervous system	Cranial nerves including smell testing and examination of larynx General neurological examination of limbs

Modified with permission from Cullen MM, Leopold DA. Disorders of smell and taste. Med Clin North Am 1999;83:57–74.

the dorsum of the tongue the taste pores remain stained blue if they are innervated. If the patient complains of dysgeusia of peripheral origin, it will be helped by local anesthetic applied to the tongue.

Assessment of salivary flow can be made subjectively by simple inspection of the secretory ducts in the floor and side of the mouth. There are three more objective methods:

1. The spit method, which requires the subject to expel saliva at regular intervals (e.g., every minute for 10 minutes).
2. In the suction method saliva is continuously aspirated for a typical period of 5 minutes.
3. In the salivette method saliva is absorbed onto a strip of paper and weighed.

The suction method is preferred by subjects and gives an approximate flow rate of about 0.5ml/minute. All these techniques are compromised by marked variability in recordings because saliva is so easily influenced by emotion, sight of food, and so forth. Patients with a dry mouth also may have a dry eye (Sjögren's syndrome), and this may be assessed by Schirmer's test. This test employs a thin strip of filter paper placed on the inferior conjunctival fornix. The degree of wetting in millimeters on each side is measured and compared to normal values.

Because taste and olfaction are so frequently confused, the sense of smell should be evaluated. The remaining cranial nerves, in particular V–XII, should be assessed. Trigeminal sensation over the anterior two-thirds and glossopharyngeal sensation over the posterior one-third of the tongue and its associated gag reflex are highly relevant. Tests of facial muscles give indirect evidence of the integrity of the chorda tympani in its proximal course. The auditory nerve should be tested because of its closeness to the nervus intermedius. Cranial nerves IX, X, and XI pass through the jugular foramen and they must also be examined. The hypoglossal nerve may be evaluated when the mouth is inspected for local disease. Neurological examination of the limbs would be relevant especially if there is question of a lesion affecting the posterior fossa.

TASTE MEASUREMENT

There are two broad categories of taste measurement: whole mouth and regional. For preliminary evaluation in a busy clinical setting the following five would be suitable as whole mouth assessment:

1. Sweet (1M sucrose).
2. Salty (1M sodium chloride).

3. Bitter (0.001M quinine hydrochloride).
4. Sour (0.032 citric acid).
5. Umami (1M monosodium glutamate).

These make colorless solutions that can be tested by asking the subject to sample 5ml without swallowing. The mouth is rinsed with distilled water and one minute should elapse between tests to avoid receptor fatigue. Clearly this will not detect lesions of a single nerve.

For more accurate whole mouth testing there are two methods. The most popular is the three-cup method. In this method subjects are presented at each trial with three drops of liquid, only one of which contains the taste stimulus—the other two contain water. A threshold measurement can be derived from this, defined as the concentration at which the subject chooses the drop containing the stimulus on either three trials in a row or on two of three trials. In the eight-cup test there are four trials with the stimulus and four without. Once more threshold assessment can be performed. Although the eight-cup method appears more sensitive the difference may relate to the fact that the mouth is rinsed out with water between test pairs whereas in the three-cup method the subject's saliva is used for cleansing the mouth.

The sense of taste can be measured on a semi-quantitative basis tested by using a taste intensity scale matched to the loudness of a 1000Hz tone. Patients are asked to identify a series of four different concentrations of salty, sweet, sour, and bitter tastes. They estimate the strength of the taste by arbitrarily assigning them a number. Varying levels of loudness of the tone are interspersed with the taste stimuli, and intensity estimates assigned to the sounds. A patient with impairment will rate a taste weaker than the sound that a healthy person rates equal.

More recent methods of whole mouth testing use either tablets or filter strips impregnated with standard stimulants. They have been found easy to use and portable. They can be self-administered and would appear to be ideal for clinical use, but neither is available commercially as yet.

The simplest regional test is electrogustometry. This uses DC anodic (H^+) stimuli from a small metallic disk placed on the tongue. In healthy people this produces a taste described variously as metallic, sour-salty, or sour. If the current is reversed so that the cathode is the stimulus the taste quality changes to sweet or bitter, but the quality of sensation is less distinct and because of this anodal stimulus is preferable. The threshold for anodal stimulus varies over the tongue but the two sides should be within 25% of each other (e.g., 8μA for the front of the tongue, 13μA for the posterior, and 20μA for the palate). In patients with Bell's palsy involving the chorda tympani the threshold for the ipsilateral anterior tongue is usually above 40μA. Electrogustometry has the advantages of being rapid, reasonably objective, and portable. More sophisticated is regional chemogustometry in which chemicals are applied to part of the tongue with a piece of filter paper, a cotton swab, or a pipette. Threshold measurement, quality, and intensity ratings can be made. A wider range of stimulants can be used by chemogustometry but the procedure is time consuming and more suited to research projects.

There have been limited efforts to develop a cortical evoked response to taste stimuli. As in olfactory evoked potentials (OEP) the trigeminal nerve is easily stimulated by mistake so the stimulant must be purely gustatory with no tactile or irritant effect on the lingual nerve. Attempts have been made using sodium chloride solution and in gaseous form, acetic acid (sour), chloroform (sweet), ammonium chloride (salty), and thujone (bitter). The cortical response is largest over the vertex as in the case of OEP and probably arises from insular cortex or medial temporal lobe regions.

In summary, the clinical evaluation of taste starts with a history and examination directed toward underlying causes. Assessment of salivary flow and oral hygiene is particularly important.

There are two methods of taste measurement: whole mouth and regional. Whole mouth techniques are traditionally of the three- or eight-cup methods. Regional assessment is simplest by electrogustometry or application of drops or filter paper containing various tastants. Cortical evoked gustometry is the most objective test but it is still under development.

SUGGESTED READING

Cullen MM, Leopold DA. Disorders of smell and taste. Med Clin North Am 1999;83:57–74.

Frank ME, Hettinger TP, Clive JM. Current trends in measuring taste. In RL Doty (ed), Handbook of Olfaction and Gustation. New York: Marcel Dekker Inc., 1995;669–688.

Jones JM, Watkins CA, Hand JS, Warren JJ, Cowen HJ. Comparison of three salivary flow rate assessment methods in an elderly population. Community Dent Oral Epidemiol 2000;28:177–184.

Kobal G. Gustatory evoked potentials in man. Electroencephalogr Clin Neurophysiol 1985;62:449–454.

Murphy C, Quinonez C, Nordin S. Reliability and validity of electrogustometry and its application to young and elderly persons. Chem Senses 1995;20: 499–503.

Investigation and Treatment of Disorders of Taste

This chapter describes taste disorders anatomically starting from the periphery to its central connections. In olfactory and hearing disorder there is a conductive component, but this is not so with taste unless one considers saliva to be the conducting medium. Inevitably there is overlap with some conditions affecting taste both centrally and peripherally. Other causes will be described, including iatrogenic disease and trauma.

Pure loss of taste is quite uncommon and apart from the lower referral rate for this condition the presence of three major afferent routes for taste from the periphery provides a back-up system in case of a single nerve failure. Even in lesions of the chorda tympani taste is sometimes preserved, possibly through an alternative pathway travelling in the mandibular division of V. Another unproven explanation relates to the so-called "release of inhibition phenomenon," whereby under normal circumstances each gustatory nerve reciprocally inhibits the other. If one taste nerve is affected, this releases its inhibitory effect and taste perception is unaltered but there may be dysgeusia. It should not be forgotten that taste perception declines with age so that reduced taste sense found in a 75-year-old may be a simple aging effect.

PERIPHERAL TASTE DISORDER

Much of this has been referred to already in the context of taste blindness and salivary function. Dysgeusia (i.e., with metallic, bitter, or salty taste) is more common than hypogeusia. Heavy smoking probably accounts for most instances of ageusia. Other common causes of ageusia relate to salivary problems. Without moisture taste cannot be appreciated. Poor mouth hygiene is often a contributor to ageusia or dysgeusia and phantogeusia is sometimes complained of especially in the presence of *Candida* infection. Inquiry should be directed toward the possibility of unhealthy teeth or dentures, gingivitis, oral thrush, cryptic tonsillitis, and chronic sialadenitis. Sjögren's syndrome is an autoimmune exocrinopathy affecting an estimated 1 million Americans that produces dry mouth and eyes. The situation is compounded further if there is associated trigeminal neuropathy involving taste afferents in the lingual nerve such that the tactile pleasure of food and drink is abolished as well. In cystic fibrosis there is hyperviscous saliva and impaired taste. Many inhabitants of nursing homes have dry mouth (xerostomia) that has been attributed to various factors including medication, mouth breathing, and dietary insufficiency. Of the latter, fiber, vitamin B6, calcium, and perhaps zinc appear to be the most important. Dry mouth is severe in patients who have received irradiation to the head or neck. This relates to both reduction of salivation from direct injury to the salivary glands and damaged taste buds. Normally taste recovers after irradiation in a few months because of the regenerative capacity of the receptor cells.

Influenzal illness can affect taste in addition to smell, and there is evidence of pathological change in the taste buds. A variety of oral and pharyngeal tumors affect taste by involving the chorda tympani or lingual nerve. The situation is often aggravated by the onset of malnutrition in such patients.

Idiopathic hypogeusia is a syndrome proposed by Henkin in which there is hypogeusia and dysgeusia, hyposmia, and dysosmia. Food has an unpleasant taste and aroma, leading to weight loss. It is alleged to be linked to zinc deficiency in the saliva but this and indeed the presence of such syndrome are not agreed universally.

Neuropathy

Taste disorder is frequent in neuropathy, especially in those with autonomic involvement. In pandys-autonomia there is dry mouth but taste is also impaired, probably because of autonomic neuropathy. In familial dysautonomia (Riley-Day syndrome) there are a reduced number of fungiform and circumvallate papillae with impaired perception of sweet and salty flavors possibly due to deficiency of BDNF. Ageusia may be the presenting symptom of AL-type amyloid and appears to be an almost universal feature in established cases. Approximately 70% of insulin-dependent (Type 1) diabetics suffer taste impairment and multivariate analysis shows that this correlates well with the presence of peripheral neuropathy. Non-insulin-dependent (Type 2) diabetics also have impairment partly reversed by correcting the blood glucose level but it is not connected with somatic or autonomic nerve function. Taste loss may be a presenting feature of Guillain-Barré syndrome where the facial nerve is regularly affected on one or both sides. In leprosy, taste impairment is extremely common, particularly in the lepromatous type where over 70% are affected.

In Bell's palsy the chorda tympani is involved typically when inflammation affects the geniculate ganglion, or more proximally as the nerve must pass through the ganglion (where its cell bodies lie) to join the nervus intermedius and reach the rostral medulla. Patients rarely complain of a taste problem but examination may show loss over the anterior two-thirds of the tongue. It is often stated that if taste loss occurs in Bell's palsy the prognosis for complete recovery is less favorable.

Metabolic and Endocrine Disease

An elevation of taste recognition threshold has been observed in renal disease and this applies particularly for sweet and sour stimuli. The mechanism of this is not known but dialysis improves the defect after at least 1 year's treatment. There were initial claims that renal dysgeusia was due to zinc deficiency but once more a claim for zinc involvement has not been substantiated. Given that patients with advanced renal disease suffer from axonal polyneuropathy a taste neuropathy analogous to diabetes would seem a possible mechanism. Individuals with liver cirrhosis occasionally report impaired taste but the mechanism is not understood. Apart from diabetes there are other endocrine diseases known to impair taste, especially thyroid-related diseases (e.g., cretinism). The latter is of considerable interest since cretins are unable to taste phenylthiocarbamide (PTC). Taste impairment has been described in about 80% cases of hypothyroidism and dysgeusia in about 40%. The taste problem does not appear to correlate with disease severity but improvement occurs with replacement treatment. The burning mouth syndrome or dysgeusia is reported in about 20% of those receiving thyroxine and treatment of thyrotoxic patients with methylthiouracil can impair taste sensitivity. Gustatory symptoms are reported in pituitary deficiency states, Cushing's syndrome as well as adrenal insufficiency.

Trauma

The chorda tympani is vulnerable to trauma in the middle ear because it is superficially placed on the upper aspect of the ear drum, hence middle ear disease or surgery thereof and head trauma are frequent causes of disorder. Because the chorda tympani has a secretomotor component to the submandibular and sublingual salivary glands as well as a gustatory component there may be a taste problem from dry mouth even if the taste fibers within it recover. The lingual nerve may be damaged from jaw trauma, difficult intubation, laryngoscopy, wisdom teeth extraction, or internal carotid artery dissection. Any of these may produce taste and common sensory loss over the anterior two-thirds of the tongue.

The jugular foramen transmits three cranial nerves—IX, X, and XI—and when they are all affected it is sometimes called Vernet's syndrome. This foramen is only rarely the site of disease such as neuroma (growing on any of these three nerves), meningioma, epidermoid, or glomus jugulare tumor. Typical symptoms are hoarse voice, nasal speech, dysphagia, and sternomastoid weakness (Color Plate 6). The glossopharyngeal nerve is usually affected, in which case taste is affected over the posterior third of the tongue.

CENTRAL TASTE DISORDER

Head injury is probably the most common central cause. The overall prevalence in head injury is approximately 0.5% and it is estimated that 6% of those with post-traumatic anosmia also have ageusia, but neither of these figures exceeds that expected by chance alone. There is little doubt that taste can be impaired after head injury, but this must be a rare occurrence and studies to date have not taken into account the prevalence rate of gustatory impairment in a noninjured population. Recovery from taste loss is said to be more likely than recovery from anosmia, perhaps because most lesions are peripheral and there are several nerves concerned with taste. It is suspected that sweet taste (chorda tympani) recovers more rapidly than bitter (glossopharyngeal nerve). Based on Sumner's literature review of 18 head-injured patients and 8 personal cases with bilateral ageusia, there is a crude relationship between duration of post-traumatic amnesia (PTA) and recovery of taste: if there is no PTA or it does not exceed 24 hours then recovery of taste can be expected within 3 months. If PTA lasts more than 24 hours, recovery may take up to 5 years. Despite this, 4 subjects with no PTA had ageusia for an unspecified time.

Brain stem damage can cause ageusia but the paucity of reports may relate to inadequate documentation of physical signs. It has been observed in unilateral medullary vascular lesions where the solitary tract or its nucleus is involved. In the lateral medullary (Wallenberg) syndrome it would be difficult on anatomical grounds to spare the solitary tract but taste loss is rarely documented. It would also be hard to avoid the superior part of the dorsal vagal nucleus (i.e., salivatory nuclei), so ipsilateral impairment of salivation should be detectable. Paramedian medullary infarcts (medial medullary syndrome) would be expected to spare the dorsolaterally situated solitary nucleus. A pontine plaque of demyelination has been found to cause ageusia in MS and there are individual cases of ageusia due to pontine or midbrain hemorrhage. There are also a few reports of vascular or demyelinating thalamic lesions causing taste loss, usually when VPMpc is damaged. Bilateral thalamotomy for Parkinson's disease has been noted to produce taste disturbance. Gustatory impairment is recognized with cortical lesions, particularly the orbitofrontal cortex, or insular zone and head injury is the most common reason for damage in these areas. In theory, a small lesion in either of these cortical regions could affect taste while sparing smell but this awaits description.

Patients with epilepsy may experience an aura of taste, although it is much less frequent than the olfactory variety. The seizure focus is located in the opercular region or amygdaloid nucleus and it is claimed to be more frequent in right hemisphere lesions.

Drugs Causing Taste Disturbance

There are an estimated 250 or more drugs that are suspected to impair taste and some of these are tabulated in Table 7-1. Because saliva is an excretory pathway for many drugs this is perhaps not surprising; they may cause taste impairment either by

Table 7-1. Drugs that may cause taste disorder*

Category of Drug	Examples
Antihelminthic	Levamisole
Antithyroid	Carbimazole, methythiouracil, propylthiouracil
Antiseptic	Chlorhexidine
Anti-inflammatory	Penicillamine, colchicine, gold salts, allopurinol, nonsteroidal anti-inflammatory drugs
Anti-mitotic	Bleomycin, alpha interferon, inter-leukin-2, methotrexate, vincristine, doxorubicin, chlorambucil, procar-bazine, cisplatin, 5-fluorouracil
Antifungals	Amphotericin B, griseofulvin
Antibiotics	Tetracycline, sulphonamides, peni-cillins, cephalosporins, ethambutol
Anti-protozoal	Metronidazole, pentamidine
Antiviral	Idoxuridine, zidovudine, didanosine, protease inhibitors (e.g., indinavir, ritonavir)
Calcium channel blocker	Nifedipine, amlodipine, diltiazem
Anti-cholinergic	Benxhexol, tricyclic antidepressants, oxybutynin *(continued)*

altering transduction mechanisms or by producing a taste of their own. Sweet appreciation is thought to be least affected by drugs because of the large number of taste buds over the anterior tongue.

Table 7-1. *continued*

Category of Drug	Examples
Diuretic	Acetazolamide, amiloride, frusemide, hydrochlorthiazide
Anti-arrhythmic	Amiodarone, procainamide, propranolol
Oral hypo-glycemic agents	Phenformin, glipizide
Anti-epileptic	Phenytoin, carbamazepine
Anti-psychotic/ antidepressant	Trifluoperazine, lithium carbonate, amitriptyline, clomipramine, paroxetine, sertraline
Drugs used in Parkinson's disease	Levodopa, pergolide, bexhexol, selegiline
Miscellaneous	Theobromine, theophylline, quinine, strychnine, sumatriptan nasal spray, metoclopramide, cimetidine, disulfiram, pesticides, lead, industrial solvents and paints

*For simplicity, only examples are given.

Hence a patient with drug-induced loss to sweet will have damage to a large number of taste buds. Many alleged associations of drugs with taste disorder are based on small numbers and are only rarely confirmed by formal testing. Certain compounds alleged to cause taste impairment might actually be causing primary smell loss. It also must be considered that the disease for which a drug is given may be the cause of taste dysfunction, not the drug itself (e.g., diabetes, thyroid disorder).

In most instances the site or mode of action is not known with certainty. Some drugs are anticholinergic and act by causing a dry mouth such as tricyclic antidepressants and anticholinergic drugs for Parkinson's disease or bladder inhibition. Antiproliferative drugs may damage the salivary acinar cells or the cell turnover in taste buds. Amiloride blocks sodium channels known to be present in taste receptors and this causes alteration in the perception of salt. Impaired taste through modification of taste receptor sodium channels may be the mechanism underlying side effects from anti-epileptic drugs such as phenytoin and carbamazepine. The antiseptic chlorhexidine is also thought to alter taste in this manner. Antineoplastic and antimicrobial drugs that disrupt DNA or protein synthesis (e.g., procarbazine, griseofulvin) can damage taste by reducing the rate of turnover of taste receptor cells. Certain bitter-tasting compounds including caffeine, theobromine, theophylline, quinine, and strychnine are known to alter second messenger systems (e.g., GTP-dependent cAMP synthesis) in the taste receptor and thereby interfere with bitter appreciation. Sulphydryl-containing drugs such as penicillamine, 5-thiopyridoxine, and captopril disturb taste perhaps through their ability to chelate zinc or they may simply be excreted in saliva.

Toxins and Pollutants

Less is known about taste disturbance from pollution compared to smell loss. There are probably more causes relating to taste than smell loss because of the excretory ability of saliva, although little is known about the excretory properties of Bowman's glands. Employees having repeated contact with pesticides such as agricultural workers may report a persistent bitter or metallic taste in the mouth. A garlic-like odor is characteristic of organophosphorus exposure and may be accompanied by other complaints such as hypersalivation, small pupils, muscle twitching, or psychiatric problems. Sweet metallic taste has been reported by workers cutting brass pipes ("metal fume fever") and in silver jewelry workers because of lead poisoning. Industrial solvents vaporize readily and are more likely to affect smell than taste, but reduced taste has been noted by printers. Painters are also susceptible, especially when solvent rather than water-based paint is used. Ciguatera poisoning and cobra or rattlesnake bites have been associated with temporary or prolonged disorder of taste, probably because of their ability to interfere with ionic channels in the taste bud. According to Indian folklore, if a patient has been bitten by a snake of unknown variety and cannot detect the burning of chili sauce in the mouth, then he or she has been bitten by a cobra.

Miscellaneous Causes

Patients suffering from depression report taste disorder often relating to anticholinergic side effects of their medication, and those with schizophrenia occasionally develop gustatory hallucinations or taste impairment that likewise is in part an unwanted effect of their drug therapy. Rarely, patients with multiple sclerosis develop impairment of taste during relapse or even at presentation.

Patients with HIV infection frequently complain of disturbed taste (and smell). This problem appears to be related to the disease per se as well as the effect of antiviral medication (Table 7-2).

The burning mouth syndrome is a multifactorial disorder affecting chiefly postmenopausal women. It may also trouble those with diabetes, Sjögren's syndrome, Parkinson's disease, pernicious anemia, dry mouth, or depression. Patients complain of a burning pain chiefly in the anterior two-thirds of the tongue, lips, and anterior hard palate. There is persistent dysgeusia and altered taste perception. Whether the

Table 7-2. Main diseases associated with loss of taste

Disease Process	Variety
Tumors	Middle ear (cholesteatoma), jugular foramen tumor (glomus jugulare)
Trauma	Chorda tympani (petrous bone fracture), lingual or glossopharyngeal nerve (neck injury), cortical trauma: insular or orbitofrontal cortex
Surgical procedure	Bilateral thalamotomy, laryngectomy, neck radiation, middle ear surgery, tracheal intubation
Vascular disorder	Lateral medullary syndrome, pontine hemorrhage, internal carotid artery dissection
Systemic disease	Diabetes (types I & II), cystic fibrosis, renal failure, familial dysautonomia, primary amyloid, Cushing's disease, hypopituitarism, Addison's disease, cretinism, cranial arteritis, Sjögren's syndrome
Infection	Bell's palsy, viral encephalitis, influenza, leprosy, periodontitis, glossitis, Guillain-Barré syndrome, AIDS
Deficiency states	Niacin (B3), vitamin A, zinc, B12
Psychiatric	Depression, schizophrenia
Developmental	Congenital facial hypoplasia
Miscellaneous	Smoking, drug side effects, aging, multiple sclerosis, Parkinson's disease, high altitude exposure, severe blood loss, snake bite (cobra or rattlesnake)

mechanism is peripherally or centrally mediated is unknown and many doubt it has an organic basis. Most likely the condition is multifactorial with some cases having an organic basis, especially in disease known to cause trigeminal neuropathy (e.g., diabetes or Sjögren's syndrome).

INVESTIGATION OF TASTE DISORDER

Investigation must start with a history and examination. For outpatient testing, the basic 5 tastants are appropriate (i.e., sucrose, saline, quinine, citric acid, and monosodium glutamate) or electrogustometry for simple regional testing. The sense of smell must also be evaluated using, for example, the 12-odor International UPSIT or sniffin' sticks. A blood screen should be performed, testing in particular the blood count (for anemia, drug effects), sedimentation rate (vasculitic disease, malignancy), B12 and folate level (nutritional state), glucose (diabetes and pituitary disease), thyroid function (myxedema), electrolytes (renal disease, Addison's or Cushing's disease), liver function tests (cirrhosis), and autoimmune tests (Sjögren's disease). Further investigation depends on complexity and whether there is a question of malingering, as may be the case in compensation claims. If cranial nerve VII is affected a thorough examination of the outer and middle ear is required, possibly supplemented by computed tomography (CT) or magnetic resonance imaging (MRI) scan of the petrous temporal bone. If there is a suspected neurological disorder affecting the brain stem or cortex (e.g., vascular, neoplastic, or traumatic) then MRI of the brain is required. Disorder of cranial nerves IX, X, or XI requires MRI of the posterior fossa, possibly supplemented by special views of the jugular foramen. MRI of the brain or neck is in general the procedure of choice as it has better overall sensitivity particularly for intracerebral lesions. For good resolution of bone (e.g., erosion or fracture) a CT scan is preferable.

TREATMENT OF TASTE DISORDER

The main drug that has been tried is zinc, but this should be given only where there is good evidence of deficiency, which is a very rare situation. Despite this, zinc salts are regularly prescribed out of therapeutic desperation if nothing else. For all other cases treatment is directed toward the underlying problem. There needs to be a thorough examination of the mouth and pharynx for evidence of infection. If the patient is troubled by dysgeusia or phantogeusia there is more likelihood of a local problem in the mouth. *Candida* infection is easily eradicated with an antifungal mouthwash (e.g., Nystatin).

A history of Bell's palsy or ear or neck surgery would lead one to suspect damage to the chorda tympani, although repair of this nerve is rarely attempted. An artificial saliva such as Xerolube may help those with xerostomia. Pilocarpine, the cholinergic drug, promotes salivary flow and is worth trying in these patients. The initial dose of 5mg four times daily has been found to alleviate the dry mouth associated with radiation to the head and neck region. Patients with dysgeusia as part of the burning mouth syndrome may be helped by application of topical anesthetic (e.g., Dyclonine 1.0%) as a mouthwash. Antidepressants or anti-epileptic drugs may be tried for this syndrome. In theory, it should be possible to help those with familial dysautonomia by treatment with the suspected missing growth factor, BDNF. If there is damage to a peripheral nerve concerned with taste it has been speculated that nerve growth factor NT3 might assist recovery.

A drug history is very relevant and reference should be made to Table 7-1. Even if the drug is not listed, a trial of withdrawal would be appropriate. If these causes are eliminated then imaging of the head should be considered.

GENERAL ADVICE FOR THOSE WITH GUSTATORY PROBLEMS

To compensate for the bland taste of food some patients eat excessively, put on weight, and consume more sugar, salt, and spice. They should be advised against this and persuaded to measure spices and herbs added to food and compensate by increasing the odor and appearance of food where possible. High salt intake may be harmful, especially in someone hypertensive, and excess sugar will obviously aggravate diabetes or obesity. Counseling from a dietician is advisable. Wine tasters, food tasters, and chefs will all be at particular disadvantage if they lose their sense of taste and a career change would be hard to avoid. Some find it difficult to come to terms with ageusia and need frequent counseling. Contact with lay societies specializing in smell and taste disorder should be considered (see Appendix).

MEDICOLEGAL ASPECTS

There are relatively few claims for personal or industrial injury due to taste loss. Those commanding the highest awards are usually engaged in the food

and drink industry. It is essential that there is in-
formed consent given by all patients who undergo
middle ear or neck surgery because of the risk of
damage to the chorda tympani or lingual nerve.

As in the case of anosmia, the courts will wish
to satisfy themselves on several counts:

- That trauma or industrial exposure can produce ageusia.
- That there was no evidence of ageusia before
  the episode.
- That local causes of ageusia have been
  excluded.
- That there is no sign of amplification of symptoms or frank malingering.
- That the prognosis for recovery is based on
  reasoned assessment.

As mentioned, in Sumner's survey of 18 head-
injured patients there is a crude relationship between
duration of PTA and recovery of taste. These figures
are based on so few patients they may well be unreli-
able, but there is nothing else available at present.

Some taste complaints attributed to pollutants
are simply a result of the sensory properties of the
pollutants themselves rather than direct pathological change in the taste receptor or neural pathway
and recovery is to be expected once the person is re-

moved from the workplace. Persons exposed to pollutants may be taking or have received medication that can affect taste sense or they may be suffering from coexisting disease known to alter gustation. It is important to quantify the degree of loss, and for this, referral to a specialist center or clinic is essential, especially where the claimant is suspected to be fabricating the taste problem.

The overall approach is similar to that concerning anosmia claims. Head injury rarely causes ageusia but if there has been a blow to the head, even trivial in nature, brain imaging (preferably by MRI) would be justified. Particular attention must be paid to the insula, orbitofrontal cortex, and temporal lobes. Functional imaging would be ideal in problematic cases. There are few examples of industrial gas or chemical exposure in association with ageusia but organophosphates, paint solvents, selenium, and other sulphur-containing chemicals have been incriminated. The threshold limit volume (TLV) or equivalent may provide a useful guide to the magnitude of exposure.

The detection of malingering in ageusic individuals is a major problem and is once more best solved in specialist centers. Threshold and identification tests are the most important initial procedures. Suspicion would be aroused if the subject claimed to detect no taste for all substances irrespective of concentration. There is crude taste appreciation from lingual nerve somatosensory fibers so that an ageusic will be able to report something even if it is just trigeminally mediated burning or irritation. As in the case of smell loss, the method of magnitude estimation compares the relationship between concentration and perceived intensity. The log of these parameters should produce a straight line. Someone with pollutant exposure has a flat slope (i.e., large increases of concentration are required to produce small increments in perceived intensity). A nonlinear relationship would arouse suspicion. The recording of taste-evoked cortical responses would be an ideal and objective approach, but this procedure is still under development.

The impact of taste loss on a wine taster or chef, for example, will command a major award as a career change will be essential. Even for those whose occupation does not depend on it, taste disturbance will have an important effect on the quality of life. It is likely that minor gastrointestinal ailments will result from hypogeusia, although there are no specific studies of this. There is a conspicuous lack of literature and guidance for ageusia claims, particularly its prognosis for recovery, but it is usually stated that taste impairment recovers better than smell loss.

In summary, taste disorder can be arbitrarily divided into peripheral and central components. The major peripheral cause is dry mouth secondary to poor hygiene. The most common neuropathy to affect taste is Bell's palsy, but diabetics and those with other metabolic and endocrine disease also suffer. The most frequent central cause is head injury with vascular and compressive lesions rare events. Numerous drugs are implicated in ageusia, some of which relate to known molecular mechanisms. Burning mouth syndrome is a common, poorly understood gustatory disorder seen most often in postmenopausal women. Treatment of taste problems should be directed to the underlying cause and empirical use of zinc salts is rarely effective and cannot be justified. General dietary and nutritional advice should be offered, particularly to the elderly, while those whose career depends on taste appreciation should have employment counseling.

SUGGESTED READING

Costanzo RM, DiNardo LJ, Zasler ND. Head injury and taste. In RL Doty (ed), Handbook of Olfaction and Gustation. New York: Marcel Dekker Inc., 1995: 775–784.

Fera MAD, Mott AE, Frank ME. Iatrogenic causes of taste disturbances: radiation therapy, surgery and medication. In RL Doty (ed), Handbook of Olfaction and Gustation. New York: Marcel Dekker Inc., 1995:785–792.

Henkin RI. Drug-induced taste and smell disorders. Incidence, mechanisms and management related primarily to treatment of sensory receptor dysfunction. Drug Safety 1994;11:318–377.

Smell and Taste Centers and Suppliers of Smell and Taste Apparatus

MAIN SMELL AND TASTE CENTERS IN THE UNITED STATES

Chemoreception Perception Laboratory
University of California, San Diego
9500 Gilman Drive
La Jolla, CA 92093-0957

Clinical Olfactory Research Center
State University of New York Health Science Center
Syracuse College of Medicine
750 East Adams Street
Syracuse, NY 13210

Connecticut Chemosensory Clinical
    Research Center
University of Connecticut Health Center
263 Farmington Avenue
Farmington, CT 06030-3705

MCV Smell and Taste Clinic
Medical College of Virginia
Virginia Commonwealth University
P.O. Box 980551
Richmond, VA 23298-0551

Monell Chemical Senses Center
3500 Market Street
Philadelphia, PA 19104-3308

National Institutes of Health
NIH Building 31, Room 3C-35
31 Center Drive, MSC 2320
Bethesda, MD 20892-2320

Rocky Mountain Taste and Smell Center
University of Colorado Health Science Center
4200 East 9th Avenue
Denver, CO 80262

San Diego Nasal Dysfunction Clinic
University of California, San Diego, Medical Center
9350 Campus Point Drive
La Jolla, CA 92037

Taste and Smell Clinic
5125 MacArthur Boulevard, Suite 20
Washington, DC 20016

University of Cincinnati Taste and Smell Center
University of Cincinnati College of Medicine
222 Piedmont Avenue
Cincinnati, OH 45219

University of Pennsylvania Smell and Taste Center
Hospital of the University of Pennsylvania
3400 Spruce Street
Philadelphia, PA 19104-4283

MAIN SMELL AND TASTE CENTERS
IN EUROPE

Common Cold Centre
Cardiff University
Museum Avenue, POB 911
Cardiff, CF1 3US Wales, United Kingdom

Department of ORL
Central Hospital
S-54185 Skövde, Sweden

Department of Otorhinolaryngology
University of Basel
Petersgraben 4
CH 4031 Basel, Switzerland

Department of Otorhinolaryngology
University of Dresden Medical School
Fetscherstrasse 74
01307 Dresden, Germany

Department of Otorhinolaryngology
University of Vienna
Währinger Gürtel 18-20
A-1090 Wien, Austria

Department of Pharmacology
University of Erlangen-Nurenberg
Erlangen, Germany

Neurosciences et Systemes Sensoriels
CNRS ESA 5020
Et Universite Claude Bernard Lyon I
69622 Villeurbanne Cedex, France

Royal National Throat Nose and Ear Hospital
Grays Inn Road
WC1X 8DA London, England, United Kingdom

SUPPLIERS OF SMELL AND TASTE TEST APPARATUS

Sniffin' Sticks, Taste Kits, and Olfactometers
Burghart GmbH
Tinsdaler Weg 175
D-22880 Wedel, Germany
Ph.: +490 4103 800 760
Website: www.burghart.net

UPSIT (and other smell and taste testing
   apparatus)
Sensonics Inc.
P.O. Box 112
Haddon Heights, NJ 08035
Ph.: 856-547-7702
Website: www.smelltest.com

Index

Page numbers followed by "t" indicate tables; "f" indicate figures.